Nutrition Hacks
The Truth

25 Years of Experience in 160 pages

Dr. John Fitzgerald, DC

Copyright © 2014 by John Fitzgerald

All rights reserved.

ISBN-13: 978-1496156631
ISBN-10: 1496156633

DISCLAIMER

This book is NOT a replacement for advice from your doctor. Show this book to your doctor and come up with a plan with your doctor to implement the strategies covered in this book.

CONTENTS

1	Choosing the Right Method	Pg 1
2	Develop a Daily Routine	Pg 5
3	Jay Kordich	Pg 16
4	Raising Nitric Oxide	Pg 21
5	Make Your Own Smoothie Recipe	Pg 25
6	Coffee and CappuGreeno Recipes	Pg 28
7	Are You Tired after Lunch?	Pg 34
8	Blood Sugar Home Testing	Pg 36
9	Don't Eat Sugar	Pg 41
10	Breaking the Binge	Pg 47
11	Monitoring Results	Pg 50
12	Is a Calorie a Calorie?	Pg 56
13	5-Day Detoxification Plan	Pg 60
14	Weight Loss Plan	Pg 67
15	Pre-Fast Meal	Pg 73
16	Other Fasting Strategies	Pg 75
17	Appetite Suppression	Pg 81
18	Pulse Test for Food Sensitivities	Pg 85

19	A Constipation Fix	Pg 88
20	Don't Drink Sodas	Pg 90
21	Endurance Training	Pg 92
22	Eating After Exercise	Pg 100
23	How much Protein do I need?	Pg 102
24	Muscle Gain	Pg 111
25	Adrenal Gland Tests	Pg 114
26	What is a Superfood?	Pg 128
27	Let Your Food be Your Medicine	Pg 130
28	Stop Getting Sick So Much	Pg 139
29	High Blood Pressure and Type 2 Diabetes Protocols	Pg 142
30	Questions for Weight Loss	Pg 149
31	Start Today – Fat Loss Guide	Pg 158

1 CHOOSING THE RIGHT METHOD

This book contains information to supplement my first book *Fat Loss The Truth*. I am going to help you reach your health, weight and lifestyle goals by providing points of emphasis that assist you in living healthier and by helping you make some adjustments to the most common pitfalls that people succumb to.

For instance, I will share how I have helped my own family, friends and patients eat more fruits, vegetables and superfoods. This daily routine is something that they completely enjoy. This is despite me being fully aware that most people have failed miserably when it comes to eating foods that help them become and stay healthy.

I, along with my cousin Matt Fitzgerald, set out to create a delivery system for eating fruits, vegetables and most importantly, "superfoods." We wanted this delivery system to be a daily routine that you depend on and enjoy so much that it becomes a way of life that you look forward to. We wanted to help those people that are willing to help themselves, through some quick, easy and effective methods of getting the nutrients that they need to be healthy.

> Our method to achieve this goal is to "hide" fruits, vegetables and superfoods into delicious smoothies recipes and superfood coffee drinks (CappuGreenos) that you will enjoy and crave. These recipes are so good you won't even realize you are eating something loaded with superfoods.

At this point in my life, I have been making fruit and vegetable juice with a juice machine and green smoothies for 22 years. I have a lot of experience doing it and know how to make these health drinks taste like a dessert. (We have put up a website to share these recipes so you can start utilizing them to benefit your health right away).

What methods should I use?

As with most things in life, there are many methods that can be used to try to achieve a result. If you truly understand the underlying principle that you want to achieve, you can pick the best and most effective method more easily.

For instance, in my first book called *Fat Loss The Truth*, I explained that the primary principle to achieving weight loss is lowering the calories (energy) that you consume. Then I explained that cutting your calories by eating fewer meals is the method that most people find easiest to follow for a long-term solution to maintain a healthy body weight.

I have done a lot of counseling with people that have previously lost weight through many different dieting methods but couldn't maintain what they were doing and gained all the weight back. They then came to me to learn about a different method for lifelong weight loss.

==The problem with their failed attempt was usually this; they used a short-term method and expected a long-term result.==

If you do not completely enjoy what you are doing in regards to the type of food that you eat, the frequency at which you eat and the amount of exercise you are doing to achieve your goals, you will inevitably fail with long-term results.

For example, I have had many people come to me saying that they eliminated carbs to achieve weight loss but then gained the weight back. I usually say something like, "Really? Do you like carbs?"

"Yes, I love them"

"So you eliminated foods that you love, how did that work out for you?"

"I lost weight but I couldn't stick with it and gained back more weight than I originally lost"

Some diet gurus look at short-term results and display before and after pictures all over their books and websites. It is frustrating for me to look at these pictures because I know the truth. I know that most of these people did not stay in the same shape as the "after" picture. Most of these people gained all the weight back and more.

I have also done a lot of counseling with women that do fitness/physique competitions. These are the women who do bodybuilding without putting on the large amounts of muscle.

They get extremely lean for the competition and their pictures in magazines display them in this extremely lean form. They do not stay in this lean form for very long. It is just for the competition. The problem is that most of these women used a method to get lean that is extremely hard to follow. After the competition is over, the girls end up heavier than where they started.

After a few competitions, they appear "chunky" and get depressed. They realize they used a method to get lean that is short term and they cannot stick with it long term. They come to me for a long-term solution to get lean and stay looking good compared to getting extremely lean for a short period of time and then looking chunky the rest of the time.

This is where daily routines come into play. Having daily routines that support long term success is crucial and that is why the next chapter is called "Develop a Daily Routine."

2 DEVELOP A DAILY ROUTINE

One of the easiest things that I have done to benefit my health and to keep my weight in check is to pick a couple of activities that I enjoy and incorporate them into my daily routine. These activities may not seem like much when viewed by themselves, but the key to seeing the benefits from them is that they are enjoyable and easy to implement in my everyday life.

My examples are:

1. Walking
2. Superfood Smoothies
3. 5 Tibetan Rites

Walking

To start every day, I walk on my treadmill at a very slow pace (2 mph). I drink 2 cups of coffee, check my emails and surf the internet. This is a time that I look forward to. I start my day with some physical activity, get caught up on current events and organize my thoughts and plan of action for the day.

I don't view this time as a chore at all. If I was making myself go run in the morning, it would soon become boring and I would not likely stick to it. I have used pedometers to measure how many steps I take in a day and I find that when I walk slowly while drinking my morning coffee and surfing the internet, it is an easy, efficient way to increase the activity in my day.

I could just as easily sit and drink my morning coffee, but I really do enjoy the slow walk. Plus, walking does a better job of waking me up and getting me going in the morning. Remember, this is a slow easy walk that isn't draining to me, mentally or physically.

Superfood Smoothies

My second activity is drinking a superfood smoothie for lunch. I can't say enough good things about doing this. I am eating a low calorie lunch that is packed full of superfoods, which help me feel and look better. The smoothies are easy to make, taste great and I don't feel like taking a nap in the middle of the day from eating a big lunch. As is the case with walking, I really enjoy the smoothie and look forward to the treat of this tasty lunch.

If I were making myself eat something that I didn't like, only because it was "good" for me, I would probably not stick with it for very long, no matter how many benefits I derive from it.

So here is what I have accomplished with these two rituals. I am getting in physical activity rather I have time to actually exercise later in the day or not. I am eating fruits, vegetables, and superfoods that help to keep me healthy.

Finally, keep in mind, not all habits are bad. It is just as easy to develop a routine from habits that are healthy, fun and beneficial. Not to mention, you are much more likely to stick with a routine that YOU truly enjoy, not just what others tell you that you "should" be doing.

5 Tibetan Rites

Dr. Vern Pierce first told me about the 5 Tibetan Rites back in 1992. Dr. Pierce was a guest speaker at the Chiropractic College I was enrolled at. He said that he gave his patients a small book, which was an instruction manual for the 5 Tibetan Rites. According to him, these exercises helped his patients get better faster and assisted with the chiropractic adjustments he was giving them.

The 5 Tibetan Rites are five yoga-type bends supposedly designed to balance your vortexes (Spinning energy centers in your body). They are said to have been used by Tibetan monks for hundreds of years (Maybe even a couple thousand years) and have the benefit of balancing the chakras of your body.

I read the book and started doing the 5 Tibetan Rites every morning when I woke up. My neck and back was all jacked up from playing football and I noticed that the 5 Tibetan Rites helped me feel better. They also seemed to give me more energy. I continued this for the next 16 years. Then when I went through a bunch of stress in my late 30's, I stopped doing them for some reason. Around the time I turned 44 years old, I read an article about the 5 Tibetan Rites and immediately started doing them again. I noticed a difference right away so I added them back into my daily routine.

I typically do them when I am halfway done with my first cup of coffee.

Each rite is performed 21 times. You may have to start by doing fewer repetitions and work your way up. I have a description below, but I encourage you to do an internet search for the 5 Tibetan Rites where you will find many videos of people actually doing the rites, demonstrating the proper form for each movement.

Rite One

Stand up with your arms out straight and palms facing down. Spin clockwise and breathe in and out while doing so. Start slow as you may get dizzy.

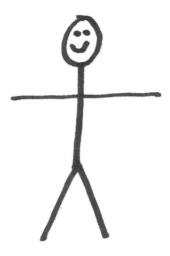

Rite Two

This is basically lifting up your head and legs together while breathing deeply. Lie on the floor on your back. Palms down next to your butt. Raise your head up and lift both legs up to perpendicular or a little further. Keep your legs straight the whole time. Breathe in as you lift your legs and exhale as you lower them.

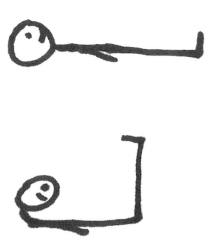

Rite Three

Kneel on the floor and keep your torso erect. Put your palms on the back of your legs right below your butt. Bend your head forward and then bend your head back as far as it can go while arching your spine backwards. Breathe deeply on the arch and exhale when you return to the starting position. Keep your toes curled under rather than flat on the ground.

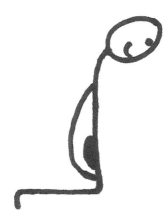

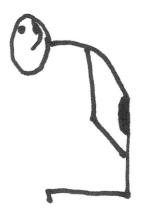

I should have mentioned this earlier. Make sure you do these rites in order. It has something to do with balancing the vortexes in a specific sequence. At least that is what a Tibetan monk said and who am I to question a Tibetan monk.

In case you are wondering if I paid a famous artist a bunch of money for these drawings, put your mind at ease, because I am the artist behind these images. Yes, I took pictures. I didn't think they were that easy to follow so I drew these stick figures. My drawings were so bad that we had to use them.

Rite Four

Sit on the floor with your legs straight out in front of you. Place your palms on the floor on each side of your hips. Bend your head forward and then all the way back as you lift up your torso, hips and knees. All that will be touching in the top position is your palms and feet and you will be in a tabletop position. Breathe in as you rise up and exhale as you lower back down.

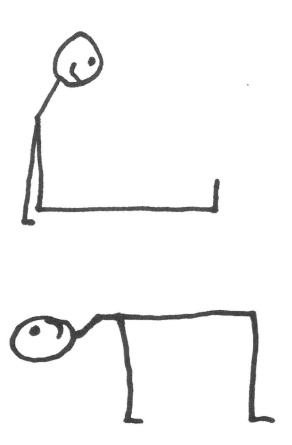

Rite Five

This is basically going from the yoga position downward dog to cobra. Put your palms and feet on the floor with your butt in the air. You will look like an inverted "V", which is called downward dog in yoga lingo. Keep your arms and legs straight while you lower your hips to the ground (cobra position). The only exception is, when you lower your hips, keep your toes curled. Breathe in on the way up and exhale on the way down.

These explanations are kind of hard to follow just reading them and pictures are a little bit of help. However, watching a short video on the internet is really easy to follow and that is why I recommend you do that now.

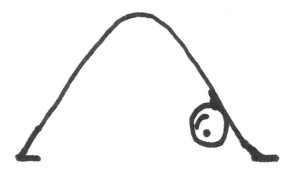

Nutrition Hacks The Truth

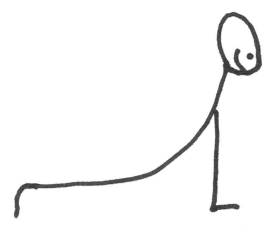

3 JAY KORDICH

So why do I write this chapter you ask? I guess, because it is nice to give credit to some people that actually deserve it.

I learned to juice fruits and vegetables from Jay Kordich. He gave me so much applicable knowledge and he changed the way I thought about food. Jay made me realize that food is medicine and eating the right food is the most powerful thing that you can do to benefit your overall health.

In the "Make Your Own Smoothie Recipe" and "CappuGreeno and Coffee Recipes" chapters, I give some instructions on how I make smoothies to incorporate fruits, vegetables and superfoods into my diet. This brief chapter is a brief acknowledgement of the man who gave me the foundation to do it.

I think what I said in this interview with Jay and Linda below, reveals my appreciation of their work.

Jay & Linda: John, we really enjoyed your book *Fat Loss The Truth*. It is a great book for losing weight and we strongly recommend it for everyone. We wanted to do a quick interview with you because you have endorsed us since you saw Jay speak around 1991.

Dr. John Fitzgerald: I was researching how to help my father with cancer and came to the conclusion that juicing would be highly beneficial. In 1991, I went with Julie, who is now my wife, to watch Jay put on a presentation in Cedar Rapids, Iowa.

Our first sip of juice was a carrot and apple mixture that Jay made himself. We started juicing immediately and put my father on a juicing regimen. It all worked well just as Jay had said it would.

I consider Jay a major gem within the natural healthcare industry. He has changed many lives with his information. He was a torchbearer for many years teaching about the benefits of juicing. Now the industry has spawned off many different juicers and blenders geared towards Jay's message of getting people to consume more fruits and vegetables.

Jay has not gotten the credit for his role in this, but many companies have profited largely from the information that Jay helped develop, refine and pass along to the masses. That's the way it goes right? I can relate. Before I published *Fat Loss The Truth*, it was a manual that many, many others stole from and claimed it as their own. Oh well, it all works out in the end and Jay and I have both provided lots of great information to help people.

Here is one more little tidbit that I had to add. Jay Kordich is the original "Juiceman". When I hear the term "Juiceman", I only think of Jay. I know that in later years, different businesses took that term and assigned it to other people, but that is not right. That is like assigning the name Superman to someone other than Clark Kent.

4 RAISING NITRIC OXIDE

Nitric Oxide has the chemical formula NO (Nitrogen and Oxygen). In humans and other mammals, NO is involved in many processes. It has led to Nobel Prize winning research and was named Molecule of the Year in 1992.

Nitric Oxide is made in our blood vessels and functions to dilate blood vessels resulting in increased blood flow. This causes better circulation all around the body. Think lower blood pressure, better brain and heart function and a better sex life.

Increasing NO is a dream for athletes because higher levels of NO equate to their muscles not being oxygen starved which means the athlete will have increased energy and endurance.

People living at higher altitude naturally produce more NO, which helps them avoid low oxygen blood levels. There are drugs for chest pain, such as nitroglycerine, which increase NO levels, causing blood flow to quickly increase. The drug Viagra helps erections by way of NO also. Diseases such as hardening of the arteries, diabetes and high blood pressure usually have low NO levels.

So you are getting the point by now, we do not want a low level of NO.

I tested my own Nitric Oxide levels using saliva-testing strips. I had come off of three days where I did not consume my usual lunch, which is a superfood smoothie or CappuGreeno. I primarily consumed foods that contained little to no fruits or vegetables in them. You can see from the picture that my level of Nitric Oxide was between depleted and low.

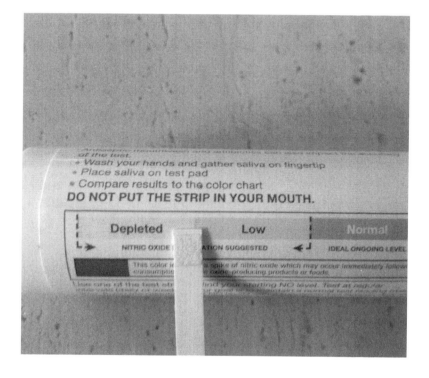

I then consumed a superfood smoothie. Actually I consumed my recipe that I have developed over the years that I call an

Energy CappuGreeno. Then I waited for 30 minutes and did the saliva test again. Here is what happened. My Nitric Oxide level was now within normal limits.

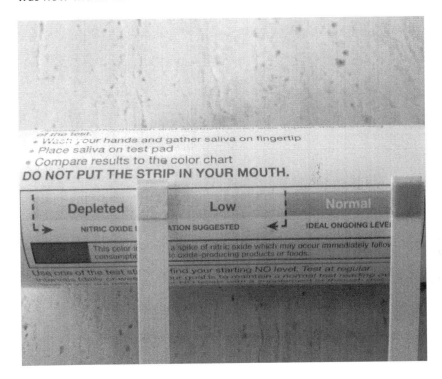

These results are why I tell athletes to consume an Energy Superfood Smoothie or an Energy CappuGreeno an hour or so before practice or games. Besides athletes, you can see how smoothies can benefit your overall health.

This is why doctors are recommending these superfood smoothies, which increase NO levels, to their patients who suffer from ailments like high blood pressure, clogged arteries and impotence.

As a side note about athletic performance, you should know that beets are probably the most advantageous ingredient, followed by dark leafy greens, such as spinach, to add into a smoothie. These ingredients boost endurance by causing a naturally occurring higher level of nitrates. The nitrates are converted into nitric oxide, which lowers the amount of oxygen needed by muscles.

In simple terms, this means that you can perform for a longer period of time without getting tired.

Here is the recipe that I mentioned earlier:

(The only difference between an Energy Superfood Smoothie and an Energy CappuGreeno is the coffee added)

Energy CappuGreeno   makes 24 ounces

170 calories per serving (12 ounces)

- 2 servings of Ancient Berry superfood mix (2 tbsp total)
- 1/2 cup coconut water
- 1/2 cup vanilla almond milk
- Coffee beans- 1 tbsp   (1 tbsp whole beans is equivalent in caffeine to 2 cups of brewed coffee)
- Vanilla Extract – 1 tsp
- Banana- 1/2 (remove the skin)
- Dates –Use 2 pitted dates
- Sea Salt – 1/8 tsp
- Vegetables:
    - Spinach – 1 cup
    - Beet ¼ (2inch diameter beet) - 20 grams
    - Fresh Mint – use 8 leaves
    - Fresh Basil – use 3 leaves
- Ice- 2 cups

5 MAKE YOUR OWN SMOOTHIE RECIPE

Eating superfoods on a regular basis is one of the best ways to stay healthy. I have found that the easiest way for my family and me to take in superfoods is to have a superfood smoothie or CappuGreeno everyday.

I have provided an overview on how to put smoothies together. However, if you want exact recipes that are really delicious, I suggest you check out the recipes at www.MyNutritionAdvisor.com

I try to get in the majority of my fruits and vegetables at lunch when I typically consume a homemade smoothie. I do this because a smoothie is lower in calories than a typical whole food meal and doesn't bog me down during the day when I am working.

If I eat a big meal at lunchtime, I don't feel like doing anything but laying around the rest of the day.

Since I want to consume food that is healthy for me, I focus on making this meal as nutritious as possible, knowing that I may not always eat fruits or vegetables at dinner. I am not perfect in what I eat and I am just being honest with myself knowing that eating perfect at each meal is not likely to happen for an extended period of time. So I put as many highly nutritious foods in my smoothie as I can.

I make these smoothies so my kids will drink them also.

The amounts of ingredients that I give below are to make enough smoothie to fill my big blender which I divide between 3 or 4 people.

These are the ingredients that I put into a smoothie.

1. I start with a liquid that includes fresh juice, coconut water or coconut milk, but most often I use vanilla almond milk.

    A. Fruit and vegetable juice that I juice myself with a juicer. I add these items:
    a cucumber or zucchini, sometimes I also add a small yellow crooked squash
    a red, orange, green or yellow bell pepper
    a bunch of greens that probably amounts to 4 to 6 cups, such as spinach, kale, escarole, bok choi, dandelion greens, parsley
    a couple of large carrots
    a beet
    an apple or pear
    a couple stalks of celery

After the juice is made, which is approximately 24 ounces, I pour it into the blender.

I will have to admit that I mostly just do the juicing when I need to use some fruits and vegetables before they go bad. Adding this step of using fresh juice typically adds about 15 minutes to the process and uses quite a bit of produce. That is why I mostly use vanilla almond milk for the liquid source.

B. Coconut water or vanilla almond milk – I only use this if I do not use the juicer.

I buy coconut water in a bottle and other times I buy a coconut and use a meat cleaver to open it. When I do, I pour the water from the coconut into the blender and then scrape out the meat of the coconut and add that to the blender also.

Sweetened vanilla almond milk tastes better than coconut water in case you are wondering. I end up using 8 – 12 ounces.

2. Superfood Mixes - I add powdered superfood blends from My Nutrition Advisor. I usually use four tablespoons.

These four tablespoons are what makes the smoothie a superfood smoothie.

3. Protein – When I add protein, I typically put in two to four tablespoons of protein. I am very picky about what protein I add. It is either a high-end

micro filtered whey isolate or a vegetable based protein.

I don't use egg, casein, or whey concentrates and I do not use any proteins with anything artificial in them including artificial sweeteners (like aspartame, acesulfame-k or sucralose).

4. A banana or avocado or both. If I have them both, I add both of them in as they add creaminess to the smoothie. If I have just one of the two, I use it. During pumpkin season, I will add cooked pumpkin in place of a banana and avocado. As you can see, I mix up the ingredients quite a bit.

5. Berries – I add some blueberries or strawberries. I probably add about ½ cup.

6. Dates - I take out the pits and add a couple dates. These are a good way to sweeten up the smoothie. The more fruit I add, the less dates I add.

7. I add some more fruit into the blender. It is usually a peach or an orange or 2 kiwis. I remove whatever needs removed before I add to the blender such as pits, skin or seeds.

8. Chocolate chips – sometimes I add a couple tablespoons when I want to make the smoothies chocolate flavor. Sometimes I add the chips at the end for 10 seconds to leave some chocolate chunks in the smoothie. I use chips that are over 50% cacao as these are better for you.

9. Ice – I fill the rest of the blender with ice. I use a lot of ice to thicken the smoothie. I also add water. The more you add, the more you thin out the smoothie.

I make this smoothie primarily based on what I have in the refrigerator. It is loaded with the healthiest foods that you can put in your body. It makes you feel better after each time you drink it.

You need a powerful blender to get this all mixed up. The popular two powerful blenders on the market are from Blendtec and Vitamix. There are also smaller volume blenders like the Nutribullet that can be used.

> Note:
> The biggest variable when throwing a bunch of ingredients in the blender and not following a recipe is that sometimes it turns out delicious and sometimes it doesn't.
>
> That is why, most of the time I follow the recipes from My Nutrition Advisor because I want a superfood smoothie or CappuGreeno that is certain to taste great.
>
> If I want recipes that are delicious and not such a mystery how they are going to turn out, I follow the recipes at www.MyNutritionAdvisor.com

6 COFFEE AND CAPPUGREENO RECIPES

A CappuGreeno is a superfood smoothie with coffee added.

Sometimes you need a kick in the nut sack and other times you need a brain freeze to have an epiphany. My epiphany came from the brain freeze (Thankfully!).

I went to a popular coffee shop and ordered an ice blended coffee drink. Halfway into the drink I had some second thoughts about what I had ordered. Mostly because of getting the most severe brain freeze I have ever had. The thing is, I make my own iced superfood smoothies nearly everyday because they are incredibly healthy and I love the taste and how they make me feel and here I was sitting on a planter in an outdoor shopping center, squinting with one eye shut from a brain freeze, as I stared at this iced coffee drink.

Now for the epiphany; As my brain thawed and my thoughts clarified, I realized that this drink all sugar and additives compared to the smoothies with coffee that I make for myself and my smoothies taste better. Right as this thought went through my mind I noticed that I had an aftertaste in my mouth from the sugar and chemical mixture in this drink. I started smacking my lips and tongue thinking I needed some water to get this taste out of my mouth.

Then I had another thought. How many calories am I consuming with this drink? Are these ingredients healthy or unhealthy? I pulled out my phone and looked it up on the internet. Over 600 calories of what I would say is a bunch of unhealthy garbage.

Holy Cow is that right? Yes it is. This realization just pushed me over the edge. I threw the rest of the drink away. I came to the conclusion that the CappuGreenos (superfood smoothies with coffee) I make myself contain way less calories than these desert coffee drinks. Plus the CappuGreenos are loaded with the healthiest superfoods on the planet. Superfoods that slash your cancer risk, help your sex life, increase your energy, help your heart and brain etc.

Another realization popped in my head, CappuGreenos taste delicious. In fact, they taste way better than this conglomeration of sugar and chemicals that I just threw away.

The final thought to hit me, as if to say, "Duh!," was that these commercially made sugar drinks are full of chemicals. When I drink one of the superfood smoothies that I make myself I feel incredible. Energized. Healthy. Strong. I do not smack my lips together thinking I need water to wash the sugar and chemical aftertaste away. At that moment, I decided, this is the last time

I will drink one of these chemical blends of crap that these big companies are advertising. I am going to drink superfood smoothies and CappuGreenos instead.

If I am not at home and there is not a location where I can get a superfood smoothie or CappuGreeno, I will order something else that is healthy. For instance, if I want coffee, I will order black coffee rather than a blended iced coffee with milk, sugar and various chemicals. If I want something cold, I order green tea.

Coffee

Why do we add whole coffee beans directly in our smoothies?

> We want to pass along all the healthy benefits of the coffee bean and we believe the CappuGreenos taste better when using the whole bean. Also, by using the whole bean, we create a time-release effect. When the whole beans are broken apart into small pieces by the blades in the blender, caffeine is released. Over a couple hours, the small pieces of beans will be digested into your system and more caffeine will be released. This is the coffee drink that keeps on giving.

When coffee beans were discovered, they were eaten for energy. Later on, people learned to brew coffee. Eating coffee beans has the same effects as drinking coffee.

An average cup of coffee is made from approximately 25 beans and contains 75 mg of caffeine. So the brewed value of each bean is about 3 mg. However, when you eat the bean, the amount is a little higher according to some sources. I am not exact on these numbers so I will give you an approximation.

One tablespoon contains approximately 50 coffee beans. I can make it strong and put 1.5 tablespoons of coffee beans into a 24-ounce CappuGreeno, which is approximately 75 coffee beans. Based on the information we have, 75 coffee beans contain approximately 225 mg of caffeine, which is equal to three cups of coffee. That is a lot of coffee per CappuGreeno. Adding more coffee beans than this ruins the taste so I usually recommend one tablespoon of coffee beans for a 24-ounce CappuGreeno for the best taste to caffeine ratio.

Recipes

Here is a CappuGreeno recipe for each Superfood mix. Note that there are a bunch more recipes on MyNutritionAdvisor.com and I have included a recipe for the Ancient Berry mix called the Energy CappuGreeno in the "Raising Nitric Oxide" chapter.

Mint Chocolate Chunk CappuGreeno   makes 24 ounces

240 calories per serving (12 ounces)

- 2 servings of Ancient Greens superfood mix (2 tbsp total)
- 1 cup vanilla almond milk
- 1/4 cup water
- Coffee beans- 1 tbsp
- Peppermint Extract – 1/4 tsp
- Banana- 1/2 (remove the skin)
- Dates - Use 2 large pitted dates
- Spinach or Kale - 1 cup
- Mango (frozen) - 1/2 cup
- Ice- 1 cup
- After blending do a last step to add chunks at the end. Add Dark Chocolate Chips – 2 tbsp. Pulse blender multiple times to break chocolate chips to desired size.

Chocolate Almond CappuGreeno   makes 24 ounces

200 calories per serving (12 ounces)

- 2 servings of Ancient Chocolate superfood mix (2 tbsp total)
- 1 cup vanilla almond milk
- 1/4 cup water
- Coffee beans- 1 tbsp
- Almond Extract – 1/2 tsp
- Dark Chocolate Chips- 1 tbsp
- Raisins – 3 tbsp
- Spinach or Kale - 1 cup
- Carrots – 1/4 cup
- Almonds - 1/8 cup
- Sea salt – 1/8 tsp

- Ice- 1.5 cups

Cinnamint CappuGreeno   makes 24 ounces

210 calories per serving (12 ounces)

- 2 servings of Ancient Delight superfood mix (2 tbsp total)
- 1 cup vanilla almond milk
- 1/4 cup water
- Coffee beans- 1 tbsp
- Vanilla Extract – 1/2 tsp
- Cinnamon – 1/4 tsp
- Dark Chocolate Chips- 1 tbsp
- Banana- 1/2 (remove the skin)
- Dates - Use 2 large pitted dates
- Spinach or Kale – 1/2 cup
- Carrots – 1/4 cup
- Fresh Mint – use 8 leaves
- Fresh Basil – use 3 leaves
- Sea salt – 1/8 tsp
- Ice- 1.5 cups

7 ARE YOU TIRED AFTER LUNCH?

This is a common complaint. People eat a "traditional" heavy food lunch of pizza, a sandwich or some other "whole" food and then go back to work. About an hour later, they are so tired that their production at work drastically drops.

My office used to be close to a Mexican restaurant where I would frequently get asked to lunch meetings. I would get back to my office and about 3 PM, I would crash. I would be so tired that it was all I could do to make it through the rest of the day without taking a nap.

Now I make it a point to not eat a heavy lunch unless I am done working for the day.

On days that I am fasting I can easily work all day long with plenty of energy. On days that I am not fasting, I drink a superfood smoothie or CappuGreeno for lunch, which gives me energy without the side effects of an afternoon crash.

During the day, when I am working, I want to be productive and attentive, so I need to be full of energy. If I eat a heavy meal, I lose my productivity and want to take a nap.

I like the idea of taking in the healthiest foods on the planet for lunch and then at the end of the day, when I am done working, I eat a heavier meal. I find that I am more productive when I structure my meals like this and I enjoy each meal more.

In addition to how effective this strategy has been for me, many clients have also given me positive feedback on their results. Give it a try and decide for yourself. I am confident that you will experience the same improvements in productivity that I and thousands of others have. Eat a smoothie for lunch and watch your energy soar into the evening as you avoid the afternoon slump.

8 BLOOD SUGAR HOME TESTING

After people read *Fat Loss The Truth*, I got a lot of questions on how to test blood sugar levels with a glucometer.

A glucometer is a small little machine that measures blood sugar. They are cheap and can be purchased at many stores as well as on the internet. You prick your finger and put a drop of blood on a test strip that goes into the glucometer, which gives you a read out of your blood sugar level.

There is a margin of error of 10% with glucometers. They are used to get a pattern of results. That means, if your glucometer reads 100, it could really be anything from 90 to 110.

Here is a pretty standard protocol to test your blood sugar.

1. Fast for 12 or more hours and check your blood sugar in the morning. You can drink a little water but nothing else. Do not exercise before the test. (A lot of doctors want to know what the blood sugar level is after fasting for 12 hours. Diabetes is considered to have a blood

sugar of 126 and above after fasting for 12 hours. Just so you know, there is a lot more to explain with diabetes and since this book isn't about diabetes, I will stop here with the explanation)
2. Test again before lunch
3. Eat lunch (something normal for you)
4. Test 1 hour after lunch
5. Test 2 hours after lunch
6. Test 3 hours after lunch

For the next couple days, write down the readings and what you ate.

The readings below are considered ideal are: (I do not use the "normal" reference ranges because they are not tight enough to provide the most advantages for long term health, instead I use "optimal" ranges)

1. Fast for 12 hours = below 86 mg/dl (Ideal is between 70 and 86)
2. 1 hour after a meal = below 140 mg/dl
3. 2 hours after a meal = below 120 mg/dl
4. 3 hours after a meal = back to what it was before you ate (depending on what and how much you ate, this can vary quite a bit)

Ideally, your blood sugar shouldn't go above 140. If it does, you should avoid, or eat less of, the food that caused it.

Here is some testing that I did on myself: (I only do this for a brief time period because I got tired of sticking myself with the needle to provide an example for you. I did eat a few widely differing foods and calorie amounts to provide a more interesting sample)

2:30 PM Superfood Smoothie 300 calories

4:30 PM 2 hours after eating blood sugar is 75

5:30 PM Pizza, Chocolate 1695 calories

6:30 PM 1 hour after eating blood sugar is 99

7:30 PM 2 hours after eating blood sugar is 93

8:30 PM 3 hours after eating blood sugar is 97

9:30 PM 4 hours after eating blood sugar is 110

10:30 PM 5 hours after eating blood sugar is 101

7:30 AM 14 hours after eating blood sugar is 85

7:30 to 8:30 I went through my morning routine, which is drinking 2 cups of black coffee with cinnamon sprinkled on top while walking on the treadmill for an hour. This is not an exercise type of speed walking. It is walking slowly at a speed between 1.5 and 2.0 while I am going through emails and surfing the internet. I find this to be relaxing while at the same time waking me up for the day.

8:30 AM 15 hours after eating blood sugar is 92

2:30 PM 21 hours after eating blood sugar is 77

2:30 PM Superfood Smoothie 300 calories

4:30 PM 2 hours after eating blood sugar is 87

Notice that my blood sugar is dropping into the "optimal" range. After a larger meal with more calories eaten, it takes longer for the blood sugar to get to the "optimal" range than after a smaller calorie meal.

Another example:

Here is another real life example that I took from some of my client files. I have had many, many people track their blood sugar levels.

18 hours after eating blood sugar is 94

24 hours after eating blood sugar is 90

27 hours after eating blood sugar is 83

Food eaten: salami, cheese, crackers, guacamole, corn chips, 2 cookies, and 3 glasses red wine

3 hours after eating after blood sugar is 111

18 hours after eating blood sugar is 91

24 hours after eating blood sugar is 75

Food eaten: Waldorf salad, salami, cheese, crackers, corn chips, and salsa

3 hours after eating blood sugar is 108

16 hours after eating blood sugar is 91

18 hours after eating blood sugar is 93

Food eaten: salami, cheese, crackers, corn chips, and bean dip

1 hour after eating blood sugar is 109

Food eaten: trail mix with nuts and dried fruit

3 hours after eating blood sugar is 90

19 hours after eating blood sugar is 90

In this example, the person's blood sugar readings were not bad. However, they will improve even more and drop more frequently into the optimal levels with time.

For instance, he had just started using my fasting protocols a few months ago and he will continue to improve with continued use of the fasting protocols. His body weight will also likely drop another 5 to 10 percent, which will help also. He typically has one CappuGreeno per day on a normal day, which was not illustrated in the above example.

My last point is that he has also just started taking nutritional supplements that I recommended to him after doing some nutritional testing. These will be beneficial as well.

9 DON'T EAT SUGAR

Processed Sugar is NOT your friend!

What should your doctor fix first?

Some of the best doctors in the country are known to focus on the big picture with patients. When focusing on the big picture, you must first correct the patient's digestion, stress response, and blood sugar regulation.

For instance, a patient comes in and wants to increase their hormone levels, but they have horrible digestion and higher blood sugar levels than they should have. You are not going to truly help this patient get the results they want unless you help fix their digestion and blood sugar levels first.

If a patient has high blood sugar levels, they are likely to also have problems with the hormones estrogen and/or testosterone. So how are you going to fix hormone problems if you don't first address the blood sugar levels?

Chronic disease costs 75% of the money spent on health care. Here is the thing; almost all chronic diseases are a result of high blood sugar, digestion and stress. That is why the best doctors work on fixing these three problems in all their patients first.

Sugar and Insulin

The more we put pure sugar into our body, the harder it is on our bodies. The more food is processed, the faster sugar gets into our bodies and the more our bodies have to adjust to this.

When people consume too much sugar, their cells start to put up a resistance. The cells resist by down regulating (kind of like turning off) the amount of insulin receptor sites.

This means less sugar is able to travel into the cells, which means the sugar remains in the blood causing a higher level of blood sugar. There will also be a high level of insulin in the blood. (Insulin is a hormone that transports sugar into cells to keep the sugar level in the blood in a specific range).

This is not good. The arteries will start to become blocked with plaque and will deprive the heart of blood which causes heart attacks.

When I refer to eating sugar, I am also talking about the foods that turn quickly into sugar such as refined carbs.

Calories Matter

In my first book, *Fat Loss The Truth*, I pointed out that the most important thing with fat loss is calories and the easiest way to lower calories is to skip meals. You should have already read the first book and be familiar with the strategies on how to skip meals. If you haven't read it, make sure you do, as you will learn much more reading both books.

Back to the lesson

Insulin has many jobs that it cannot do if blood sugar is high. For instance, insulin carries magnesium into the cell. When the insulin receptor sites are blocked, people have low levels of magnesium in their cells. I have seen this problem over and over. There is a chronic problem with people having low magnesium. Due to poor farming practices that do not replace all the essential minerals back into the soil, people are chronically low in many important minerals such as magnesium and zinc.

To make matters worse, eating a bunch of sugar lowers your magnesium levels. On the other hand, a study showed that taking magnesium decreased fasting insulin levels and improved 60 genes that are related to metabolism and inflammation. You can find the study here in case you are wondering: Am J Clin Nutr February 2011 vol. 93

By the way, a standard blood test is not a good way to measure total body magnesium. Your body will keep a tight range of magnesium in the blood while your cells are highly deficient.

You can get a test done with a specialty lab (Spectracell) that measures the level of magnesium in white blood cells. I run these tests frequently because they give a more accurate reading of the true nutritional status in your body.

So why is this important? Magnesium is necessary for energy production. An athlete low in magnesium will not be able to perform at their personal top level because energy production can't be perfect with low magnesium. Here is the kicker; almost every athlete I have ever tested has been low in magnesium.

Magnesium is also necessary for a healthy heart and normal blood pressure. A high level of insulin in the blood also causes fluid retention, which can increase blood pressure and make you feel bloated. Remember that this is all from eating sugar. I personally feel bloated from all the water retention whenever I eat a bunch of dessert, which raises my blood sugar and causes a rise in insulin.

Fasting is the fastest and most effective way to lower blood sugar as I stated in *Fat Loss The Truth*.

Most will agree that fasting insulin levels should be below 10 and a better level is below 6. If insulin levels are above 10, insulin resistance is well under way.

To lower your insulin levels, start following the protocols for skipping meals in the first book. To make fasting even more effective, you should stop eating sugar and refined carbs. Weight lifting also helps.

Use the pulse test in this book to eliminate any food sensitivities you may have. This may also have an effect.

Lastly, make sure you look at the examples in the chapter called, "Blood Sugar Home Testing". Notice that after consuming a superfood smoothie, my blood sugar did not elevate nearly as much as a large meal of pizza. The superfood smoothies are lower calorie meals that consist of fruits, vegetables and super foods.

What about Fruit?

My short answer is that fruit is good for you and stop worrying about it.

There are people who believe that fruit is bad for you because it contains sugar. Here is what is being overlooked. Fruit contains things that actually help to improve your blood sugar levels, even though fruit contains sugar.

For instance, fruit contains phytonutrients that have a large number of health benefits. One benefit is the improvement of insulin sensitivity.

Fruit contains fiber, which slows down how fast sugar enters the blood. Fiber also nourishes the good bacteria in the gut. This good bacteria helps to improve insulin sensitivity.

When people eat fruit, their blood sugar levels do not respond like when they eat pure, refined sugar or processed foods containing sugar. I have monitored blood sugar levels on many overweight people and on myself for many years. I have seen some of the most significant improvements in blood sugar when superfood smoothies were incorporated into the diet. Actually, I can't think of anything that has been more beneficial to the overall health of my patients and my family than superfood smoothies and fruit is an ingredient in almost all of my superfood smoothie recipes.

10 BREAKING THE BINGE

Your weight will likely fluctuate within a particular range on a day to day basis. When it starts getting towards the top of that range or exceeds the range that you have established, it is important to immediately take action and get yourself back to a weight where you feel comfortable and healthy.

One of the components that I knew I needed to include in this book, is providing a simple and easy to follow method to get back on track after going on a binge. Everyone binges and some of us with more addictive personalities will tend to binge more often then others.

As I write this I am coming off a bad binge of stuffing myself with my trigger foods, pizza and chocolate. This has been going on and off for the last month. I have had company and we were out partying on the Las Vegas Strip. There has been excessive partying, eating, drinking and a lack of sleep. I weighed myself this morning and was 10 pounds higher than what I am comfortable with. What makes it even worse is that I was already near the top of my range when the binge started.

How did this happen? Is it because on December 21, 2012 the world is supposed to end so I just decided to let loose? No, I didn't really believe that so I couldn't blame it on the world ending. It would be a convenient excuse though. How about this reason? I stopped tracking my calorie intake and weighing myself. Yes, this is probably the reason I gained weight. I didn't have the constant feedback to keep myself in check, so I went off the reservation and my weight crept up.

I better get this under control right now or I am going to end up fat. I know that many of you have said the same thing, but what can you do to turn your eating habits around to lose the weight you just put on?

You have probably said things like "starting tomorrow, I am going to just eat salad" or "I am going to only eat (fill in the blank) for the next month".

Then about halfway through the next day, you cannot stop thinking about all the different foods you want. So you fail and go get a cheeseburger or something similar that you are craving.

What can you do to make a change that you will actually stick with you ask? Pick the foods you like and eat them. Yeah, you heard me right.

The meals I pick are:
1. Superfood Smoothies and CappuGreenos
2. Cheeseburgers
3. Steak and salad
4. Bacon, cheese, onion and red bell pepper omlette

These are foods that I love to eat and I do not feel deprived eating them.

I pick these foods because these are not my trigger foods. I define trigger foods as something you eat that you cannot portion control. These foods lead to an overeating of large amounts of calories. My trigger foods are pizza, ice cream, cake and milk chocolate. However, I am going to be eating dark chocolate frequently because it satisfies me, I like it, it is good for me and I typically don't grossly overeat it.

Most of the time, I will have a superfood smoothie for lunch and one of these other foods for dinner and I am very satisfied. Then a few times per week, I will just have 1 meal in the day. If I feel in the mood for some other food, I will have it. There isn't a hard line on exactly what I will and will not eat.

The other things that I do are things to help me mentally. I start listening to hypnosis tapes again each night when I go to bed. I find that these tapes really focus me and from time to time getting refocused helps.

Another thing that I do to help me mentally is start reading *Fat Loss The Truth* again. Obviously, nobody knows that book better than I do, because I wrote it. However, when I read the book, it gets me focused again.

Ok, here we go. I am breaking the binge starting today. Remember what Apollo Creed told Rocky, "There is no tomorrow". In other words, start today.

11 MONITORING RESULTS

Here are some additional pointers when it comes to monitoring yourself or a client. Writing down what you are tracking makes a big difference. It helps to keep you accountable and allows you to analyze what you are doing.

Weighing:

Weigh yourself everyday at the same time and then average the numbers for the week. Compare the average for the week with the average from last week to truly see how you are doing.

Here is how I recommend doing it. Weigh yourself right after you wake up in the morning. Get up, go to the bathroom and then step onto the scale for a reading. This will allow the weight to be taken at consistent times. One of the problems with clients being weighed and measured in your office once per week is that they usually have a different schedule each day, so the weighing times are not consistent. Also, what they eat before weighing in is not consistent each time. We fix this by having the client weigh at home at a consistent time and then compare the weekly averages.

I have a scale that syncs with my phone and keeps track of it for me, which makes the process even easier.

Calorie Tracking:

This is one of your most valuable tools.

I keep track of the calories I eat using a phone app. I would recommend trying several free ones and see which one you like.

I simply add the food that I eat each day into the phone app. and shoot for a weekly average.

If you are not losing fat you should count your calories until you do start losing fat. This is an exercise for you to see how many calories you are actually consuming.

For instance, you will find that veggies do not add up to high amounts of calories, while ice cream contains a substantial amount of calories.

Let's say that a good starting point for a man to lose weight is 1800 calories per day and for a woman would be 1200 calories per day. Divide that amount between the two meals.

A man would ideally have 2 meals per day that total less than 1800 calories for the day. A woman would keep her intake of food to less than 1200 calories per day.
If you are losing weight each week, you are on track. If you are not losing weight, simply lower the calories you are consuming. Remember this; if you are not losing weight, it is almost always because you are eating too many calories.

Tape Measurements

I have already mentioned that 1 inch on a waist measurement is equal to approximately 5 lbs of body fat. Monitor your waist measurement from week to week. If your waist drops ½ inch, you lost roughly 2.5 lbs of body fat. This is another way to monitor how your body is changing. If your scale weight did not drop, but your waist measurement dropped, you likely lost some body fat and gained some muscle.

Monitor your steps with a Pedometer:

Set a goal of how many steps you want to take in a day and make sure you get there. I have seen great results when getting at least 10,000 steps per day. I have averaged 13,000 to 15,000 steps per day over quite some time.

I tell clients that they must reach at least 10,000 step everyday. If they are at 7,000 steps and it is 7 pm, they better go for a walk or start pacing in their house to make sure they reach at least 10,000 steps for the day. Most people take around 800 to 1000 steps for every 10 minutes of walking.

One of the reasons that I walk every morning is so that I am able to reach my step total for the day.

Stagger your calorie intake:

It is better to be staggered in the amount of calories you are consuming. In other words, do not eat the same thing everyday and do not eat the exact same amount of calories everyday.

So rather than eating exactly 1200 calories every day, mix it up a bit. (Day 1) you might eat 1800 calories, (Day 2) 1100 calories and (Day 3) 700 calories. The goal is to eat 8400 calories for the week, which averages out to 1200 calories per day.

When you are using fasting for weight loss, your calorie intake is pretty much automatically staggered because on fasting days, your calorie intake will be lower.

I have seen many people that like to eat around their maintenance calories each day and then cut the calories 2 to 3 times per week by eating 1 meal on those days. For instance, let's say that maintenance calories are approximately 1650 calories per day. Sunday, Wednesday, Friday, and Saturday eat around 1650 calories per day. Monday, Tuesday and Thursday eat around 500 calories per day. You can cut down to only 1 or 2 days if you want to lose at a slower rate.

Eat a variety of foods:

Eating the same thing everyday can lead to food sensitivities. Eating the same amount of calories can allow your body to adapt a bit and can also lead to water retention.

Water Retention:

Many times people confuse their metabolism slowing down with water retention. That is because, at a certain point, your body can hold water and your scale weight will stop lowering for a period of time due to the water retention. This does not mean your metabolism has completely slowed down. It typically means that the water you are retaining is offsetting the fat lost when you weigh yourself. When you eat a larger meal, you will typically lose some, if not the majority of the retained water.

Food Sensitivities:

You can be sensitive to a food without being completely allergic to a food. Also, there are different levels of food allergies. Let's say that someone is allergic to peanuts. They will probably never be able to eat peanuts without some type of physical reaction. Some people have such high reactions that they can die from just coming in contact with the food they are allergic to.

Someone who is sensitive to a food can have a lower level reaction such as increased heart rate or an immune system response. Eating the same food too frequently for their body to handle is usually what develops the sensitivity. This does not mean that you will always develop a specific food sensitivity from eating the same food too frequently.

However, it can and does happen to many people. There are blood tests to measure food sensitivities just like there are blood tests to measure food allergies.

If the irritating food is avoided for a period of time, the food sensitivity usually goes away. Sometimes the avoidance only needs to be a couple weeks and other times it might take six months to clear up.

I will tell you how to test yourself for food sensitivities in the chapter "Pulse Test for Food Sensitivities".

12 IS A CALORIE A CALORIE?

Here are a couple of very confusing statements. "A calorie is a calorie" and "A calorie is not a calorie".

When people use these statements they are referring to something that is completely unrelated to the actual definition of a calorie. This creates confusion.

Let me clear up the confusion and be as sarcastic as I can be.

A calorie is a unit of measurement.

What are other units of measurement you ask? An inch, a mile, a gram, a gallon, etc., etc.

No one ever says, "An inch is not an inch." However, there is a lot of exaggeration when it comes to inches.

So what exactly does a calorie measure? Heat. Not how

healthy a particular food is or is not perceived to be. It is simply a measurement of heat.

Here is the simplistic definition:

A calorie is a unit of measurement used to quantify the amount of energy that foods will produce in the human body. I know we can be a lot more specific but I am trying to make this simple. Ok, Ok, I will get a little more specific.

Here is the scientific definition:

A calorie is the amount of heat needed to raise the temperature of 1 gram of water by 1 degree Celsius at normal atmospheric pressure.

Here is what a calorie is not:

It is not a type of food or a way to say that one particular food is more nutritious than another. It is not a way to say that a particular food is healthy and you cannot get fat eating that food. There are No "healthy food" calories that "magically" disappear when they enter your body.

It is not a way to say that you should become a vegetarian and stay away from meat because meat is evil. You see, when someone makes comments like these, they sound like an idiot. They may actually be an idiot if they say that a calorie is the nourishment in natural foods that makes one healthy.

How about this little gem that self-proclaimed masters of

wisdom dispense with regularity on nutrition websites. "Calories don't matter". This is one of the most idiotic statements in all of nutrition.

Here are some correct statements:

Your body requires a certain amount of energy per day. This energy is measured in calories. If you eat more calories than your body needs, the excess calories will be stored as fat. If you eat fewer calories than your body needs, you will lose weight.

Some foods contain a lot of calories and some do not.

Usually, healthy foods contain a fewer amount of calories than unhealthy foods. However, this is not always the case. For instance, raw walnuts contain a lot of calories and are healthy, while diet sodas contain very few calories and are unhealthy.

Different types of food react differently in your body. For example, protein can reduce your appetite while fructose can stimulate your appetite. Some foods are beneficial to your hormones, immune system and overall health and some are not.

If a large amount of the calories you consume come from unhealthy foods, you will be less healthy than if they come from healthy foods. Isn't that obvious?

Foods that react negatively with your hormones can cause you to gain weight quicker and lose weight slower when compared to the same amount of calories from food that react positively with your hormones.

However, calories do matter and if you consume fewer calories than your body needs, even from unhealthy foods, you will still lose weight. You can choose to make the source of calories you eat come from healthy or unhealthy foods.

You will feel and look much better if you choose healthy foods.

13 5-DAY DETOXIFICATION PLAN

We need to do certain things on a regular basis to detoxify our bodies. My daily routine contains elements that promote daily detoxification. This is an important thing to understand because it makes a massive difference in how you look and feel.

Here is one of the main reasons why we need to detoxify. According to the United States Food and Drug Administration (FDA), back in 1998, over 35% of the food tested contained pesticide residues. In 2013, 53 pesticides classified as "carcinogens" were registered for use on major crops. There is also more than 10,000 additives being used in our food supply. An average American eats about 142 pounds of additives a year. You can thank the elected officials in Washington DC for this. If you voted for Democrats or Republicans, you likely supported this being done to our food supply.

So what are some common symptoms of toxin buildup you ask?

Allergic reactions, backaches, blood sugar problems, constipation, fatigue, headaches, hormone Issues, immune weakness, joint pains, mood changes, sinus issues, skin problems and the list goes on but I think you get the picture.

With liver detoxification there are two phases. Phase 1 occurs when the toxins within your body are activated by enzymes in your body. In Phase 2, enzymes convert these toxins into harmless, water-soluble molecules that can then be eliminated.

This detoxification process is highly dependent on vitamins, minerals and an overall good nutrition level because without these nutrients, your liver cannot clean itself. Since superfoods have the greatest nutrition levels of any foods, they strongly support detoxification.

Why did I pick five days?

There wasn't a specific medical reason for five days. It just seemed like the follow through really dropped off when I would recommend longer times for patients. I know people who do shorter programs more frequently because they like how they feel when doing a two or three day detoxification every month or two.

This detoxification plan is actually quite easy if you already incorporate my favorite eating schedule, consisting of drinking a CappuGreeno or superfood smoothie for lunch everyday and then eating a meal for dinner. The only difference is to replace the meal at dinner with a superfood smoothie.

When you incorporate a fasting time everyday into your normal eating schedule, you are already taking advantage of the most effective way to detoxify yourself. I personally do two things that help my liver detoxify itself on a daily basis. I fast approximately 18 hours between dinner and lunch the next day and I drink a CappuGreeno or superfood smoothie for lunch nearly everyday.

Follow these rules below to get the most out of this plan:

Rule 1: Choose a different superfood mix recipe for each meal. For a variety of nutrients, never do the same recipe in the same day. If you use the same superfood mix in a day, choose a different recipe.

Here are the four super food mixes:

Ancient Berry

Ancient Chocolate

Ancient Delight

Ancient Greens

It is ideal if you choose a different superfood mix for each meal. If that isn't possible on any particular day, I would vary the recipes you use with each superfood mix for each meal.

Rule 2: One of the most overlooked times of detoxification is during the fasting hours rather than the eating hours. When your body is not actively digesting food, your liver can better focus its efforts on detoxification. This is one of the many benefits of fasting on a daily basis.

To get a greater benefit from you detoxification, I recommend that you incorporate a daily fast of 18 to 24 hours. Another way to look at it is this: Consume all your superfood smoothies for the day in a six-hour window.

Rule 3: Drink water, tea or coffee. Adding a slice of things such as lemon, lime, cucumber, orange or mint leaves into the water gives it a nice flavor and adds health benefits. Drinking green, white or red teas all have health benefits. If you drink coffee, add cinnamon or make sure it is black.

Rule 4: Drink one to four smoothies per day. If you consume less calories you will lose weight faster (if that is your goal).

Here is a real example of how I did the plan:

I started this after dinner on Tuesday night and only had superfood smoothies or CappuGreenos until Sunday night.

Day 1

I ate Dinner last night (Tuesday) at 8:00 PM. I had my cousin Matt Fitzgerald in town for five days on business. (He is the business mind behind My Nutrition Advisor) We decided that I should include my detoxification plan in this book and on the website, so I decided to just go ahead and do it while I write about it. So here it goes:

7:30 AM Two cups coffee with ground cinnamon.

(15 hrs fasting) 11:00 AM Peachy Blueberry Superfood Smoothie 24 ounces (Ancient Berry)

12:00 PM Heirloom Pear Superfood Smoothie 12

ounces (Ancient Delight)

4:30 PM Peanut Butter and Jelly Superfood Smoothie 12 ounces (Ancient Chocolate). Mint Chocolate Chunk Superfood Smoothie 12 ounces (Ancient Greens)

Total ounces drank today = 60, I have been full all day and feel very good.

Day 2

9:30 AM Two cups coffee with ground cinnamon.

(19 hrs fasting) 11:30 AM Caramel Apple Superfood Smoothie 12 ounces (Ancient Delight)

1:30 PM Energy CappuGreeno 12 ounces (Ancient Berry)

5:00 PM Peanut Butter Cup Superfood Smoothie 24 ounces (Ancient Chocolate)

Total ounces drank today = 48, another good day, as I am feeling great.

Day 3

10:00 AM Two cups coffee with ground cinnamon.

(21 hrs fasting) 2:00 PM Irish Cherry Chocolate Chunk CappuGreeno 24 ounces (Ancient Berry)

5:00 PM Peanut Butter and Jelly Superfood Smoothie 24

ounces (Ancient Chocolate)

Total ounces drank today = 48, I have done a lot of detoxification protocols and none have been as easy to follow as this one.

Day 4

8:30 AM Two cups coffee with ground cinnamon.

(19 hours fasting) 12:00 PM Salted Chocolate Caramel Superfood Smoothie 24 ounces (Ancient Chocolate and Ancient Delight)

5:00 PM Chocolate Covered Cherry Superfood Smoothie 24 ounces (Ancient Berry)

Total ounces drank today = 48, I am feeling great and this has been so easy to follow.

Day 5

9:30 AM Two cups coffee with ground cinnamon.

(19 hrs fasting) 12:00 PM Salted Chocolate Chunk Superfood Smoothie 24 ounces (Ancient Chocolate)

I am going to eat a food dinner at about 5:00 PM, which will end the five-day program.

Summary

I have always felt great the whole time on this program. It is easy to follow and doesn't leave you feeling deprived.

This is also a great way to start things off when you are changing how you eat. For instance, before you start applying the fasting protocols to lose weight, do a five day detoxification program.

14 WEIGHT LOSS PLAN

In this section I go into some more detail on my favorite way to implement the methods in *Fat Loss The Truth*. I didn't want to go into too many details in that book about what foods I like to eat because I wanted to give people total freedom to apply the methods with whatever foods they chose.

One of the reasons that I didn't write about my specific dietary choices is that I get in modes where I eat certain foods for some time and then totally change everything. Just by me writing what I am eating may be enough to influence others to think they need to do the same thing, which simply is not the case.

The following plan is something that you can modify to start getting weight loss results immediately. I am going to use myself as the example because I know my exact metabolic measurements and have done this many times with both my clients and me.

My resting metabolic rate the last time I measured it was 1850 calories per day. So I have set a goal to average 1800 calories per day or lower. This number will likely fluctuate and I will be able to see how my body reacts.

I do not count exercise calories because I will likely underestimate my total calorie intake just like studies have shown people to do. I figure the underestimation of calories consumed and not counting exercise calories will likely cancel each other out.

Remember, this is not an exact science when it comes to counting calories. Rather it is a general guide that helps you learn how much food you can eat to lose, gain or maintain a body weight.

For each week, I want to do one of two things. The options are: See my average weight for the week lower and/or set a new low for my weight on at least one day of a week.

I will also be monitoring my waist measurement. Since 5 lbs of fat equals about 1 inch on a waist measurement, I would like to see my waist drop ¼ inch per week. That is equal to 1.25 lbs of fat lost. However, improvements are typically not linear between all measurement and weigh ins. Look for the good in either weight or tape measurements.

There are a few things that will help your long-term success that I want to make you aware of.

1. Your daily calories should not be reduced the same amount everyday. What is important is the amount of calories that you average for the week. That way your body never adapts to a specific amount of calories and it keeps you from feeling deprived. As a side note; if you drop your calories low enough, and eat the same amount everyday, you will still lose weight. In fact, you can lose weight rapidly doing this. However, this is very hard to maintain.
2. Don't rely on calculating exercise calories to drop weight. The important part for weight loss is reducing the amount of calories you are eating. However, exercise is very beneficial and I really like doing my daily routine of walking, which I cover in another chapter, additionally, I also like yoga. Weight lifting is also highly beneficial. I want to be clear; for long-term success, drop calorie intake to lose weight rather than creating a deficit from exercise.
3. You can easily make up for high calorie days by using fasting to achieve some low calorie days to average things out. I have personally gone through the holidays eating what ever I want and I still lost weight. You can do the same thing to achieve success.
4. It will likely help you to write down what you do everyday such as what and when you eat, what you weigh and the calorie count. Also, compare your waist measurement from week to week.

Here is my typical schedule: I just keep cycling the days. After Day 3, I start over again at Day 1, which is listed as Day 4 below.

Day 1

7:30 AM Two cups coffee with ground cinnamon. Walk slowly for one hour. Do 5 Tibetan Rites.

8:30 AM Yoga for 30 minutes

12:00 PM Superfood Smoothie = 400 calories

6:00 PM Cheeseburger, baked fries and/or salad (whatever I am hungry for) = 1250 calories

Total calories today = 1650

Day 2

7:30 AM Two cups coffee with ground cinnamon. Walk slowly for one hour. Do 5 Tibetan Rites.

8:30 AM Weightlifting for 20 minutes

(18 hrs fasting) 12:00 PM Superfood Smoothie = 500 calories

6:00 PM Steak, red wine, potatoes, mushrooms, cheese, pita bread, caprese salad = 1450 calories

Total calories today = 1950

Day 3

7:30 AM Two cups coffee with ground cinnamon. Walk slowly for one hour. Do 5 Tibetan Rites.

8:30 AM Yoga for 30 minutes

(18 hrs fasting) 12:00 PM Omelette = 650 calories (If I do less calories than this I will usually do one of the CappuGreenos as they are good at suppressing my appetite)

I will skip Dinner on this day.

Total calories today = 650

Day 4

7:30 AM Two cups coffee with ground cinnamon. Walk slowly for one hour. Do 5 Tibetan Rites.

8:30 AM Yoga for 30 minutes

(24 hours fasting) 12:00 PM Superfood Smoothie = 400 calories

6:00 PM Cheeseburger, baked fries and/or salad = 1250 calories

Total calories today = 1650

The thing to notice in this example is that Day 1 and 2 are very close to my maintenance calories. Day 3 is a lower calorie day that typically incorporates a longer fasting period that extends into day 4. Day 3 and 4 are my days that I am losing weight doing a longer fast and lower calorie intake.

How to modify the plan for yourself

The calorie counts can vary significantly, but here are some general starting points.

Women: Start at averaging 1200 calories per day for the week.

Men: Use my numbers and average 1800 calories per day for the week.

15 PRE-FAST MEAL

Many times you can make things a lot easier on yourself by slightly tweaking your approach.

I am going to fast from noon today until noon tomorrow. Here are a few things that will make this easier to do.

1. I am going to eat a meal that is approximately half of my baseline calories (BMR). My baseline is between 1900 – 2000 calories per day. So I am going to eat a meal that is approximately 950 calories.

2. This meal will consist of some protein. Protein has appetite suppressant qualities. Today, I am eating tuna salad on crackers. Not because that is the perfect meal, but rather because that is what I am hungry for and it contains protein. I frequently eat a cheeseburger before a fast because it mentally satisfies me.

3. I am not eating sugar at this meal. Sugar makes you hungrier sooner so I don't eat it before a 24 hour fast.

4. My dessert will consist of two coffee espressos with cinnamon sprinkled on top. Coffee acts as an appetite suppressant and cinnamon helps slow the rate at which food leaves the stomach and also acts to stabilize blood sugar.

16 OTHER FASTING STRATEGIES

In *Fat Loss The Truth*, I included the most effective and easy to follow fasting methods that I have used. In the last example, I give some specifics on what I have found that patients are most likely to follow through with.

Here are some other methods that you may like to utilize that are slightly different from the methods in *Fat Loss the Truth*.

1. Every other day

2. Skip a day

3. Fast off body weight

4. Juice Fast

5. Smoothie for lunch and then eat a meal for dinner. (My favorite method)

1. Every other day

There are several variations of this method and also several names.

One variation is commonly called alternate day fasting. The method that most people follow is where they free feed (eat what and how much they want) on day one and then on day two, they eat 25% of their required calories.

I am big on tracking calories with my weight loss patients. I cover it in the "Monitoring Results" chapter. You should know how many calories your body burns each day at rest, which is called the resting energy expenditure or BMR (Basal Metabolic Rate).

For instance, my body burns 2117 calories per day. I know I used another figure earlier in this book, but I just did another test and this is what came back so I will go with the updated information. This figure does not include exercise.

With this method of fasting, I would free feed on day one and then eat 2117 x 25% = 529 calories on day two. I then alternate back and forth from day one to day two. This method is simple, yet allows for variety and keeps you from feeling deprived.

I have used this method on patients and modified it for better results. Here is something that I have found to work better for some people. However, the most important thing is to follow a method that you are most likely to stick with.

Eat your resting energy expenditure amount of calories on Day one. For me, this is 2117 calories.

On Day two, eat 33% of your resting energy expenditure. For me, that would be 2117 x 33% = 706 cal.

Alternate between these two caloric totals from day to day.

On Day one, you would typically eat two meals.

On Day two, you would typically eat one meal.

2. Skip a day

This was one of the first methods of fasting that I used. It is very simple. Pick a day and don't consume any calories on that day.

The reason I use this method infrequently is that I find the difficulty level is much higher when you go a full day without eating. However, it is much easier to do it on a day where I am not at home and am busy.

Example:

Eat lunch and dinner on Monday

Do not eat Tuesday

Eat lunch and dinner on Wednesday

This was the method of fasting that Paul Bragg recommended doing once per week in his book *The Miracle of Fasting*. He also recommended skipping breakfast for a daily fast which is something that I like to do for myself and recommend to others.

3. Fast off body weight

I think this is one of the hardest methods to apply. It is hard to do mentally. Therefore, it is not a method I typically recommend. I am mentioning it here because every once in a while, I will have someone that likes this method the best. I will state again that my favorite methods are in the first book, *Fat Loss The Truth* combined with number five below.

Think of it this way; eat like a lion. Eat a big satisfying meal and then go a period of time until you eat again. I know people who have had success taking this method one step further. They don't eat again until their bodyweight is back to their pre-meal weight or lower. So they judge when to eat based off their body weight.

One last comment about this method is that body weight should not be the only factor that you pay attention to. For instance, I once had a male who weighed 185 lbs. After he achieved his goals with me, he still weighed 185 lbs. However, he had lost over three inches around his waist and dropped his body fat percentage by several percentages. He had removed body fat and replaced it with muscle and he looked terrific.

4. Juice Fast

This is not true fasting in the purest definition of the word. Fasting is when you go a period of time without taking in any calories and juice definitely has calories. Technically, this is a detoxification program rather than a fast.

I used to do a lot of juicing and juice fasts. I did so much juicing in years past that I burned out three juice machines. Now, I actually prefer to make superfood smoothies and CappuGreenos. They taste better, use less produce and the cleanup is substantially quicker. Compared to a juicer, a powerful blender is so much easier to clean. This fact alone leads to much greater follow through for myself and for my patients.

I have done a lot of juice fasting because this is what I put my father on when he got cancer. We would simply drink freshly made juice several times per day. We did not eat any solid food. We were following something called the Gerson cancer therapy.

The juices we drank were primarily vegetable based with an apple thrown in to sweeten up the flavor.

Our timelines were typically one to three days of only consuming juice. Then we would go back to consuming both juice and solid food.

5. Smoothie for lunch and then eat a meal for dinner (my favorite method)

I have used this method quite a bit. I like it and find it easy to follow. It is essentially the method from my book *Fat Loss The Truth* where I eat twice per day. I typically eat lunch and then eat dinner within six hours. I then fast until lunch the next day, which is typically 18 hours later. Sometimes I move the fasting to 20 hours and eat in a four hour window.

Since weight loss is about calorie reduction and fasting is the best way to accomplish calorie reduction, fasting remains to be the basis of the program I follow.

I make a superfood smoothie or CappuGreeno for lunch that contains about 300 - 500 calories. Note that these calories are coming from the healthiest food sources known to man. These are the type of calories that react very well within your body. In the chapter, "Is a Calorie a Calorie?," I discuss briefly how certain foods can benefit your hormones, immune system and overall health. Eating foods that contain calories from really healthy sources can really help your body optimize weight loss. The superfood smoothies and CappuGreenos provide calories from sources of foods that are highly beneficial to your body.

Let me word this another way. If you eat a 500-calorie superfood smoothie for lunch compared to 500-calorie cupcake, you will put your body in a much better position to be healthy and burn fat. However, you can still lose weight eating the 500-calorie cupcake.

Since I have such a low calorie lunch, and then a regular dinner, I have further reduced the calories I have eaten. This leads to faster weight loss and makes it easier to maintain my current weight if I eat large dinners containing higher calorie levels.

If I am not losing weight, it is because I am eating too much for dinner. When someone tells me this scenario, I simply have him or her eat less for dinner. I usually recommend more protein and vegetables for dinner, which fills them up more, is lower in calories and helps with hunger. They find it easier to fast until lunch the next day.

17 Appetite Suppression

These are the different ways I look at appetite suppression:

1. To take something before you eat so that you eat less at your meal.

2. To take something after your meal so that the meal keeps you satisfied longer.

3. To take something in between meals so that you have less hunger.

Each one of these has a viable method to help you reduce hunger. I give you a solution for each one below.

1. This method addresses the problem of eating too much at each meal.

    Have you ever eaten a large meal really quickly and then about half an hour after you finished eating, you feel fuller than when you actually stopped eating? That is because it takes 20 minutes for the stomach hormones that act as messengers, to tell your brain that you should stop eating. When you consumed a bunch of food too quickly, you actually ate to fast for your "fullness alerting hormones" to work.

There are methods to assist your stomach hormones in getting your brain the messages that you have had enough food. The methods I use are to take either ½ to 1 teaspoon of My Nutrition Advisor superfood mix (I usually use the Super Berry or Super Chocolate), essential fatty acids or fiber with a glass of water about 20 minutes before you start eating your meal.

This allows the "fullness alerting hormones" a chance to start the clock on alerting your brain that you are eating before you begin with the actual meal. Try it. It really works. The dosage I typically recommend is three pills of either fiber or essential fatty acids (fish oil or flax seed oil). One tablespoon of chia seeds also works well and contains both fiber and essential fatty acids. Chia seeds are also in the My Nutrition Advisor superfood mixes. My favorite is to use a teaspoon of either Super Chocolate or Super Berry 20 minutes before the meal.

2. This method addresses the problem of getting hungry shortly after you just got done eating.

The goal here is to slow down the rate at which food leaves your stomach and small intestines. This helps reduce hunger. The strategies I use are summed up in three words: Protein, coffee and cinnamon.

Protein takes longer to digest than carbs, so make sure what you are eating has protein in it. Protein reduces hunger.

If it is lunchtime and I am going to skip dinner, I find a cup of coffee or an espresso works well. Caffeine is an appetite suppressant. I typically wouldn't use this strategy at dinner because I don't want the caffeine to keep me up at night.

Cinnamon slows the rate at which food empties the stomach. Sprinkle some cinnamon directly into your coffee. One last strategy is to take ½ to 1 teaspoon of the My Nutrition Advisor superfood mix, Ancient Delight, immediately after your meal. This mix contains cinnamon and will make the overall meal more nutritious and satisfying.

3. This method addresses the problem of wanting to snack between meals.

   In between meals, there are things that you can do to reduce hunger:
   Peppermint oil, cha de bugre, coffee, physical activity, water

   Peppermint oil has many beneficial qualities. One of them happens to be appetite suppression. One drop on your tongue is enough to do the trick. I do not use peppermint extract for this. I use 100% pure peppermint essential oil.

   Cha de bugre (sha day boo grey) is an herb that has appetite suppressant qualities. I like the supplement called Fat Burn by My Nutrition Advisor taken between meals.

   Drink coffee. As I said earlier, caffeine is an appetite suppressant. However, I would keep it below 4 cups per day. Once you go above 4 cups, you can and typically do start to negatively affect your adrenal glands. I personally find that 2 cups per day is best for me. Sometimes I do another cup after lunch once or twice per week.

Get up and move. Physical activity reduces hunger. Walk, do housework, exercise, go run errands. The exception to this is doing cardio exercise, such as jogging, which tends to make you hungry. The worst thing you can do is sit on your ass watching TV.

Drink water. Dehydration will make you feel hungry when all you really need to do is hydrate yourself.

18 PULSE TEST FOR FOOD SENSITIVITIES

This test is used to check for sensitivities to things such as food and supplements.

(Certain medications can make this test NOT work properly. For instance, calcium channel blockers and beta-blockers both alter the heart rate, which can alter this test)

This is a modified version of the test that was developed by Dr. Coca, an allergist who had been board certified for over 40 years.

By way of trial and error he determined that the body could determine if something was healthy or unhealthy. When you put something in your mouth, your nervous system reacts to the substance and one of the ways to check this reaction was by taking your pulse.

Here is how to do the test:

1. Take your pulse for a full 60 seconds to establish a baseline reading. Actually count your pulse for 60 seconds rather than a shortened amount of time. Put your reading in the "Pulse Before" column.

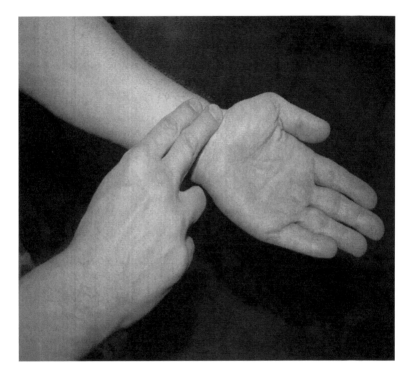

2. Put a supplement or food directly onto your tongue and hold it in your mouth for 30 seconds. Do not swallow and test only 1 thing at a time.

3. After 30 seconds with the food or supplement in your mouth, take your pulse again for another full 60 seconds while the food/supplement is still in your mouth. Record the reading in

the "Pulse After" column.

4. If you are going to test additional items, spit out whatever you just tested and start the entire process from step one. Also, remain seated the entire time. Getting up and walking around, even if it is just to spit out your prior test food, will increase your pulse. Your pulse must return to normal and then you can test another food or supplement. You may have to rinse your mouth out with water a few times and wait a couple of minutes for your pulse to return to normal.

Pulse Before   Food   Pulse After   Difference

(If your pulse increases by 4 or more, the substance is considered to be causing a stressful reaction. The higher the pulse increases the more stressful the substance is to you at this time. You may want to avoid that substance for a few weeks and test again. Many times the substance will stop being stressful if it is avoided for a period of time)

19 A CONSTIPATION FIX

The best solution that I have ever used for my patients to help constipation is consuming a superfood smoothie everyday.

I decided to write this chapter after I was in Iowa for three weeks on business. I was working on a plan to teach dieticians how to make superfood smoothies during cooking classes and seminars. In one particular meeting, I was asked if the smoothies help constipation. Before I was asked the question, I just assumed everyone knew that these smoothies are a remarkable solution for many people suffering from constipation. Then I realized that so many more people could be helped if they were made aware of this benefit.

A couple of days later while still in Iowa, a 60-year-old woman who I will call, "Bonnie," asked me for help. She said that she always feels bad. Bonnie said that she has low energy levels, sleeps poorly at night, which makes her tired all day long and has suffered from constipation for as long as she can remember.

I showed her how to make a Chocolate CappuGreeno and an

Energy CappuGreeno. I instructed her to enjoy a CappuGreeno at breakfast and/or lunch. I also told her she should pick a superfood smoothie without coffee in it if she does one for dinner. I told her that she would likely settle in to doing one smoothie per day.

Two weeks later, she called and said that she has drank at least one smoothie everyday and it has changed her life. She was so happy. She said that the constipation and low energy levels that she suffered from were immediately corrected and that within a week she was sleeping through the night.

Matt Fitzgerald and I joked about naming a specific smoothie "Colon Blow" or "Ass Cleaner". However, when it comes down to it, we really didn't need to make a specific smoothie for constipation because the superfood smoothie and CappuGreeno recipes we have already work well for constipation.

20 DON'T DRINK SODAS

One of the most harmful things you can consume is soda. It stimulates hunger, screws up the hormone insulin and is highly acidic, which can lead to many diseases. Multibillion-dollar companies promote soda, but don't get confused, as it is not good for you even in the slightest.

I commonly hear obese people tell me that they drink a 2-liter bottle of diet soda per day. They are confused and think it is ok to drink, since the soda is diet. If you really want to lose weight, stop drinking soda and switch to water or green tea.

The study below shows that all soda contributes to weight gain and diet soda actually causes more weight gain than regular soda.

Drinking soda is related to weight gain

For diet soft-drink drinkers, the risk of becoming overweight or obese was:

36.5% for up to 1/2 can each day
37.5% for 1/2 to one can each day
54.5% for 1 to 2 cans each day
57.1% for more than 2 cans each day.

For regular soft-drink drinkers, the risk of becoming overweight or obese was:
26% for up to 1/2 can each day
30.4% for 1/2 to one can each day
32.8% for 1 to 2 cans each day
47.2% for more than 2 cans each day.

Fowler, S.P. 65th Annual Scientific Sessions, American Diabetes Association, San Diego, June 10-14, 2005

A good alternative to soda is naturally flavored sparkling mineral water.

There were typically only a few foods that I used to like to drink soda with. However, after switching to sparkling mineral water, I prefer it to soda because it is not so sweet and doesn't increase your thirst for water like soda does. For instance, when I have pizza, instead of having a soda with it, I cut up a lemon or lime, put the slices in a glass of ice and add sparkling mineral water. Sometimes I even add several mint leaves. It tastes great and is good for you. Following my suggestion just a few times will create a healthy habit, rather than a destructive habit like soda.

21 ENDURANCE TRAINING

Short Answer: Train in the fasted state for best results. Your body will make adaptations when you train in the fasted state. There are more beneficial improvements in things that are important to athletes such as VO2Max and muscle glycogen levels.

The Kenyans, who pretty much have ruled the sport of long distance running, train in the fasted state. Also, this practice is now being used by many of the top athletes in endurance sports. At first this may sound strange, but the more you look into it, the more sense it makes.

Increased Energy

Training in the fasted state means that you are training with low amounts of glycogen (sugar that your body uses for energy) in your muscles. This forces your body to adapt to this state. Your body adapts to this so well that it actually rebounds and you have higher resting levels of muscle glycogen. This is a good thing since muscles that have more energy stored in them can do more work.

Increased Oxygen

Another benefit of training in the fasted state is an increase in VO2Max, which is the maximal oxygen uptake. Obviously, it is better to be able to take in more oxygen than less oxygen.

The competition

When it comes to the actual competition, endurance athletes typically compete in the fed state. So the guidelines for optimal competition performance: compete in the fed state and train in the fasted state.

Interesting Research

In my first book, *Fat Loss the Truth*, I generally recommend fasting 18 to 24 hours rather then multiple days on end. I did come across some research of athletic performance when people fasted for longer periods of time and how it affected athletic performance.

(My Notes: For most people, fasting will not make a noticeable difference, even after 3.5 days)

Influence of a 3.5 day fast on physical performance.

Eur J Appl Physiol Occup Physiol. 1987;56(4):428-32.

Eight young men were tested for strength, anaerobic capacity and aerobic endurance in a post absorptive state and after a 3.5 day fast.

Strength was tested both isokinetically and isometrically. Anaerobic capacity was evaluated by having subjects perform 50 rapidly repeated isokinetic contractions of the elbow flexors at 3.14 rad x s-1.

Aerobic endurance was measured as time to volitional fatigue during a cycle ergometer exercise at 45% VO2max. Measures of VO2, VE, heart rate, and ratings of perceived exertion were obtained prior to and during the cycle exercise.

The 3.5 day fast did not influence isometric strength, anaerobic capacity or aerobic endurance.

Isokinetic strength was significantly reduced (approximately 10%) at both velocities. VO2, VE and perceived exertion were not affected by fasting. Fasting significantly increased heart rate during exercise but not at rest.

It was concluded that there are minimal impairments in physical performance parameters measured here as a result of a 3.5 day fast.

(My Notes: This study done by the US Army showed that there wasn't a difference with soldiers exercising to exhaustion even if they haven't eaten for 3.5 days)

Influence of fasting on carbohydrate and fat metabolism during rest and exercise in men.

US Army Research Institute of Environmental Medicine, Natick, Massachusetts 01760. J Appl Physiol. 1988 May;64(5):1923-9.

Metabolic effects of an overnight fast (post absorptive state, PA) or a 3.5-day fast (fasted state, F) were compared in eight healthy young men at rest and during exercise to exhaustion at 45% maximum O2 uptake.

Glucose rate of appearance (Ra) and disappearance (Rd) were calculated from plasma glucose enrichment during a primed, continuous infusion of [6,6-2H]glucose. Serum substrates and insulin levels were measured and glycogen content of the vastus lateralis was determined in biopsies taken before and after exercise.

At rest, whole-body glucose flux (determined by the deuterated tracer) and carbohydrate oxidation (determined from respiratory exchange ratio) were lower in F than PA, but muscle glycogen levels were similar.

During exercise, glucose flux, whole-body carbohydrate oxidation, and the rate of muscle glycogen utilization were significantly lower during the fast. In the PA state, glucose Ra and Rd increased together throughout exercise.

However, in the F state Ra exceeded Rd during the 1st h of exercise, causing an increase in plasma glucose to levels similar to those of the PA state. The increase in glucose flux was markedly less throughout F exercise. Lower carbohydrate utilization in the F state was accompanied by higher circulating fatty acids and ketone bodies, lower plasma insulin levels, and the maintenance of physical performance reflected by similar time to exhaustion.

Just some friendly advice from me if you are a competing athlete:

If you do your endurance training while fasted, you will burn more fat for energy than you would if you were not fasting. However, Fasting is not an effective strategy for an endurance competition such as a race.

Using some fasting strategies during training may help you perform better on competition day. Competition day is not the time to fast. Fasting for 27 hours and longer will shorten the time it takes an athlete to exercise to exhaustion.

This is further seen in more extreme endurance competitions such as marathons and triathlons where athletes intake calories during the event.

(My Notes: If you are competing to win a race, Fasting is not effective for endurance type exercise. On the other hand, if you want to burn fat, training in the fasted state is the way to go. Blood sugar levels remained the same whether the athlete fasted or not, so that is not a concern. These were highly fit athletes that were training at a professional level, which a small percentage of people would ever be able to do)

Running endurance in 27-hour fasted humans.

Center for Health Promotion, Loma Linda University, California 92350. J Appl Physiol. 1987 Dec;63(6):2502-9.

Nine male marathon runners were exercised to exhaustion to determine the effects of a 27-hour fast on endurance performance.

Each subject completed two exercise tests at the same treadmill speed (set at 70% maximal O2 uptake), one following a 27-hour fast and one 3 hours after a pre-exercise meal, in random order.

Fasting caused a 44.7 +/- 5.8% (SE) decrease in endurance performance. Blood, muscle, psychological, and ventilatory data were examined to determine the cause of the decreased performance.

Fasting caused significant increases in O2 uptake (9.3 +/- 2.0%), heart rate (8.4 +/- 2.4%), and rating of perceived exertion, ventilation, and psychological fatigue, evident within the first 60 min of exercise.

There were no differences in plasma glucose (sugar) or epinephrine levels. Muscle glycogen degraded at the same rate despite lower respiratory exchange ratio and elevated free fatty acid levels, which may partially explain the elevated O2 uptake.

Lactate, insulin, and norepinephrine were all increased in the fasted test. The increase in norepinephrine, the diameter of type I muscle fibers, and ending insulin levels were correlated with endurance time in the fasted state. Fatigue in endurance running for 27-hour fasted humans appears to be related to a combination of physiological, psychological, metabolic, and hormonal changes.

> **(My Notes: Endurance performance was decreased with a 36 hour fast)**

Effects of a 36-hour fast on human endurance and substrate utilization.

Exercise Physiology Laboratory, University of California, Berkeley 94720. J Appl Physiol. 1990 Nov;69(5):1849-55.

To determine if prolonged fasting affects substrate utilization and endurance time, seven trained men exercised to exhaustion on a cycle ergometer at 50% maximum oxygen consumption (VO2max) in an overnight-fasted [postabsorptive (PA)] state and after a 36-hour fast (F).

Fasting produced significant elevations in the resting concentrations of blood free fatty acids (F vs. PA, respectively, a 107% increase), beta-hydroxybutyrate (beta-OH, a 1,270% increase), and glycerol (a 200% increase), with a significant decline in glucose (79.79 vs. 98.88 mg/dl, a 19% decrease).

Exercise in the F trial increased FFA, decreased glucose, and significantly elevated beta-OH and glycerol over the PA trial. There was no difference in blood glucose concentration between trials at exhaustion.

However, F produced a significant decrement in exercise endurance time compared with the PA trial (88.9 +/- 18.3 vs. 144.4 +/- 22.6 min, F vs. PA, a 38% decrease).

Based on the respiratory exchange ratio, fasting led to a greater utilization of lipids during rest and exercise. It was concluded that 1) a 36-hour fast significantly altered substrate utilization at rest and throughout exercise to exhaustion, 2) glucose levels do not appear to be the single determinant of time to exhaustion in submaximal exercise, and 3) despite the apparent sparing of carbohydrate utilization with the 36-hour fast, endurance performance was significantly decreased.

22 EATING AFTER EXERCISE

Quick Overview: Athletes can benefit from post workout nutrition, if you are a regular person who wants to get lean and stay lean, don't bother.

Eating right after a workout:

What has been popularized by the media is the notion that there is a magical period right after you exercise where amino acids (protein) can get into your muscles. There are mixed thoughts about this strategy. Many experts believe this to be speculative at best.

To make this really simple, here is a quick overview.

If you have one or more days rest between intense workouts, you will not likely need to worry about post workout nutrition.

If you are an athlete and will be working out again that same day or the next day, you could benefit from post workout nutrition.

One strategy that has been followed is to have some type of high glycemic carb drink (aka sugar) after training. This is not really necessary, unless you will be training again in the next 24 hours in some type of endurance type of training.

If you eat in a normal manner, it takes about 48 hours for your glycogen stores to be fully replaced.

I figure that the healthiest drink that I can have is one of My Nutrition Advisor's superfood smoothies for a post workout drink. If I was playing a sport again in high school or college, a superfood smoothie after practice would help me recover for practice the next day and it would also give me a bunch of superfoods to help keep me healthy during the season. That would have been great compared to the unhealthy ice cream milkshakes that I commonly made after an exhausting practice.

23 HOW MUCH PROTEIN DO I NEED?

This is a topic that is highly overdone with a constant supply of misinformation. If you listen to the advertisements, you will believe that it is necessary to eat a large amount of protein to burn fat, build muscle and in general live healthy.

Just so you know, the average recommended amount of protein for people is approximately 50 grams per day. Studies show that even for men who are lifting weights and gaining muscle, 120 grams of protein is plenty.

The recommended daily allowance (RDA) for protein is 0.8 grams of protein for every 2.2 lbs of bodyweight per day. For example: 150 lbs bodyweight divided by 2.2 x 0.8 = 54 grams

There is another recommendation based upon how much lean body mass you have, how active you are and how many calories you consume. It is called the Acceptable Macronutrient Distribution Range (AMDR). The protein recommendations range from 10 – 35% of total daily calories you are eating, rather than dictating the amount of calories and protein you actually need. So as you can see, this is also more of a guideline than an actual scientific based exact measurement.

Protein is essential

Most foods contain at least some protein but the amounts can vary significantly. For instance, an apple would have a lower amount of protein than a steak. I am sure you already knew that.

Protein is made up of amino acids strung together, in a particular order. When you eat a protein, your digestion process breaks the protein back down to amino acids, which are absolutely necessary to live.

Your body uses amino acids to build necessary things all over your body, including muscles. Amino acids are also necessary for muscle repair.

So the question is this: How much protein do we actually need?

Scientists have used several different methods to address this question and come up with a consistent answer.

One method used to measure protein necessity is called nitrogen balance, which is a measurement of nitrogen movement. This was looked at because nitrogen is involved with protein metabolism. **Nitrogen balance, which has been theorized, to relate to muscle gain or loss, in actuality has never been proven to actually be able to show muscle gain or**

muscle loss. It is common for advertisements to talk about nitrogen balance even though it just doesn't pan out when it comes to gaining muscle.

An advertisement may say something like this: You need such and such amount of protein to remain in positive nitrogen balance. Then they give you some numbers commonly between 1 to 3 grams of protein per pound of bodyweight. For instance, 150 lbs of bodyweight x 2 grams = 300 grams of protein recommended per day for a 150 lb person. In reality, measuring nitrogen balance has not proved to be a reliable marker for gaining a bunch of muscle and even a big man working out hard doesn't need more than 120 grams of protein per day.

An important point to understand is that eating more protein does not equal more muscle.

Let's say that you eat 2000 calories per day and 5% of those calories come from protein. Then you switch to a diet where you still eat 2000 calories per day but now 50% of those calories come from protein. The greater percentage of protein in your diet will not suddenly be converted to muscle. Rather the extra protein (amino acids) will be used as fuel and burned for energy.

As a side note to increasing how much protein you consume will cause your body to adapt. One of the amazing things about our bodies is the ability to constantly adapt. Your body will adapt to different types of food that you eat. A person who eats more protein is going to be able to absorb more protein. A vegetarian, who eats small amounts of protein, will likely have digestion problems if they switch to a high protein diet. However, after a month or so, there body will likely adapt and they will be able to digest the added protein.

Another interesting fact

Did you know our bodies manufacture protein? That is why some amino acids are considered essential, meaning you must get them from your diet. Your body produces non-essential amino acids.

The good bacteria in our gut called microflora, manufactures amino acids. As a function of our bodies constantly repairing themselves, these amino acids are being moved around where they are needed.

What makes big muscles?

Obviously men have larger muscles than women (mainly because of hormonal differences) also, there are genetic differences between people. One man may naturally have a lot more muscle than another man. What is known is that stressing a muscle repeatedly with heavy weights causes it to become stronger and grow. Many older adults experience the opposite of this. When they were 18 years old, they were active and playing sports. They had larger muscles and were more toned. Now they sit at a desk job and are inactive for the most part. Their muscles have shrunk and are no longer toned because they do not stress their muscles like they did when they were 18.

How much muscle can be gained with lifting weights?

Studies have shown that with 4 months of weight training, most people can gain 2 to 5 lbs of muscle. Young men may be able to double this figure if they still have high hormone levels and have not already put on muscle from lifting weights.

This goes against everything you have probably ever heard about protein requirements

One particular study indicated that lifting weights causes your muscles to adapt, which changes the amount of protein they need. Interestingly enough, long-term weightlifters muscles become so efficient that their protein needs actually drop rather than rise. I know that sounds like a complete contradiction with everything you have ever heard, but realize this; The human body and most things in nature have an incredible ability to adapt. Todd KS, Butterfield GE, Calloway DH. Nitrogen balance in men with adequate and deficient energy intake at three levels of work. J Nutr. 1984 Nov;114(11):2107-18.

It is frustrating to talk to meatheads

I recently had a guy say that taking testosterone is less than 10% of how he achieved his bodybuilder physique. He wanted me to believe that he got that unnatural amount of muscle primarily by lifting weights and drinking protein shakes. So I had to add this question and the true answer, because he was irritating me so much. So here it goes.

What do bodybuilders do differently to gain large amounts of muscle compared to a person who lifts weights, watches what they eat but only gains a little bit of muscle?

They take steroids. Pretty simple answer, but that is the answer.

You probably have not heard about the study in 1996, where 43 men who train with weights were given testosterone (steroids) and exercise. They lifted weights 3 times per week for 10 weeks and received weekly steroid injections.

They were divided into four groups.

1. Control Group did no exercise and took no steroids = gained 0 lbs of muscle
2. Group 2 did NOT exercise and did take steroids = gained 6 lbs of muscle
3. Group 3 did exercise and did NOT take steroids = gained 4.5 lbs of muscle
4. Group 4 did exercise and did take steroids = gained 13 lbs of muscle

Note: All 4 groups ate the same amount of protein, which was 0.7 grams of protein per pound of body weight (which amount to approximately 120 grams of protein per day) and approximately 16 calories per pound of body weight.

Taking 120 grams of protein per day was clearly enough for these men to gain lots of muscle.

Group 1 and 4 took the same amount of protein. Group 1 did not gain muscle, yet group 4 gained 13 lbs of muscle. This clearly indicates that protein was NOT the deciding factor with gaining muscle. What made the biggest impact gaining muscle was taking testosterone, followed by lifting weights.

Here is the study in case you are further interested: N Engl J Med. 1996 Jul 4;335(1):1-7. The effects of supraphysiologic doses of testosterone on muscle size and strength in normal men.

The same researcher who did this study did another study in 2005 with 52 men. He once again gave the men (who were in their 60's) testosterone and this time varied the dosages from 25 mg, 50 mg, 300 mg to 600 mg weekly.

The men ate around 100 grams of protein per day and around 2500 calories per day. They did not exercise and were followed for 20 weeks.

If protein were the deciding factor to how much muscle was gained, every group would have gained the same amount of muscle. However, the guys who took the largest amount of testosterone gained the largest amount of muscle. The guys taking 600 mg weekly gained 16 lbs of muscle averaging a daily protein intake of approximately 100 grams.

Here is another point to understand. Sixteen pounds was a big muscle gain to be achieved in 20 weeks. These men achieved this 16 lb muscle gain eating 100 grams of protein per day, NOT 300 grams of protein per day, like some people would want you to believe is necessary.

Another way to think of this is that eating 100 grams of protein per day did not limit these guys from gaining muscle. What limited them from gaining muscle was testosterone. The guys who took more testosterone gained more muscle and the guys who took less testosterone gained less muscle.

How much protein is too little?

A group of people who have kidney problems were put on a low protein diet. They ate 0.3 grams of protein per day per pound of bodyweight for 12 weeks. Then they did something that most people would believe increases protein need; they lifted weights. Here is what happened: they actually got stronger and their muscles got bigger lifting weights while on a low protein diet.

Should you increase carbs or protein to increase muscle?

Here is a study that was published in 2002 where 73 men participated for 8 weeks. They were put into 3 groups. All three groups followed the same workout program.

Group 1: consumed an extra 2000 calories per day, which included an extra 106 grams of protein per day. They ended up gaining 6 lbs of muscle.

Group 2: consumed an extra 2000 calories per day, which included an extra 24 grams of protein per day. They ended up gaining 7.5 lbs of muscle.

Group 3: did the same workout program but did NOT increase extra calories. They ended up gaining 3 lbs of muscle.

The two groups that significantly upped their calorie intake gained more muscle than the group that did not. The group that upped their protein intake the most did NOT gain the most amount of muscle.

There is only so much protein that your body can use to build muscle and once you go beyond that point, it really ceases to matter.

Overall what should I learn from this chapter?

1. Above 120 grams of protein eaten per day seems to have little if any benefit for those trying to gain muscle.
2. You can gain a certain amount of muscle from lifting weights.
3. You gain a lot of muscle by taking steroids.
4. Taking protein supplements do not cause you to gain a lot of muscle.

24 MUSCLE GAIN

These are the three things that one must focus on to gain muscle.

1. Lift Heavy Weights
2. Increase Calorie Intake
3. Optimize Hormones

Lift Heavy Weights

I am not going to comment on every workout routine there is and how each one differs. However, I will tell you this: pick a workout routine that includes lifting heavy weights and stick with it.

Increase Calorie Intake

Your muscles need an increase in calories (energy) to grow. I have clients track their calorie intake to get an idea of how many calories they are currently eating. There are many free phone apps to track calories. The goal is to be consistent on your calories and then on workout days add another 500 to 800 calories. (I do this by adding a superfood smoothie before or after the workout).

If you are not gaining muscle, start by upping your calorie intake 200 calories per day. If your waist is getting bigger, you are putting on body fat, which is not good. That means you are eating too many calories. If you are not tracking your calories, you will not have enough information to make adjustments to how many calories you are eating.

Remember what you learned in the last chapter, protein intake is highly overrated. It is not required for you to eat 300 grams of protein per day to gain muscle. As long as you eat 60 to 120 grams of protein per day, you are eating enough protein to gain muscle.

Optimize Hormones

It is important to optimize your hormones without shutting down your natural production of hormones. If you take steroids, testosterone or growth hormone, you will shut down your natural production of hormones. Many people shut down their natural production of hormones and have to rely on taking prescription drugs for the rest of their lives. Also, driving your hormones ridiculously high can cause a gain in muscle, but frequently comes with long term side effects.

What I use to optimize hormones is primarily velvet antler (from deer and elk antlers and is the number two ingredient in eastern medicine) and tribulus (an herb). These are safe, effective and will not shut down your natural production of hormones. Don't waste your money on cheap products, they aren't effective unless they have a high concentration of the necessary ingredients, which precludes them from being "cheap."

25 ADRENAL GLAND TESTS

This chapter contains a lot of information and you will need to be read it a few times to fully understand it. If you believe this chapter relates to you, it will provide an invaluable starting point to get yourself functioning normally again. I have changed so many lives for the better by utilizing this information.

A common problem people suffer from is weak adrenal gland function. It is so common and causes so many diverse symptoms that I decided to add this chapter.

I am focusing on giving you things that you can do at home for evaluation. These tests can completely change your health and for athletes can drastically improve how you perform.

What are the Adrenal Glands ?

First I will give an overview of the Adrenal Glands and how important they are to your overall health and performance.

The adrenal glands are located on top of the kidneys and secrete the hormones commonly known as adrenaline and cortisol.

The hormones from the adrenal cortex are necessary to live, unlike the sex hormones and hormones from other endocrine glands.

Because of this, the adrenal hormones are considered top priority by your body, and your body will wisely sacrifice functions of your reproductive organs and digestive tract in an attempt to repair your adrenals.

Each adrenal gland is made up of two parts: the outer region, called the adrenal cortex and the inner region, called the adrenal medulla.

Adrenal cortex = produces a group of hormones:

Corticosteroids: are synthesized from cholesterol and have an effect on electrolyte balance (most noticed when one feels puffy from water weight gain) and have an important effect on blood glucose concentrations.

Cortisol: control the body's use of fats, proteins, and carbohydrates, as well as exhibiting anti-inflammatory and immune system effects. Cortisol production is almost entirely controlled by adrenocorticotropic hormones (ACTH) from the anterior pituitary. ACTH also encourages the production of androgens. ACTH, in turn, is controlled by the hypothalamus through the human chemical corticotrophin-releasing factor (CRF). The cells that make CRF are believed to be in the limbic portion of the brain, indicating that CRF can be strongly affected by external stressors and emotional states of being.

Aldosterone: maintains blood volume and blood pressure.

Androgen hormones (in small amounts): play a role in the regeneration of tissue, particularly the bones, muscles, and skin, and have an effect on the development of masculine characteristics.

Adrenal Medulla = helps us deal with the physical and emotional stresses. It secretes these hormones:

Epinephrine (Adrenaline): increases our heart rate and the force of heart contractions, facilitates blood flow to the muscles and brain, causes relaxation of smooth muscles, and helps with conversion of glycogen to glucose in the liver. It is considered one of the "fight or flight" hormones.

Norepinephrine: strong vasoconstrictive effects, thus regulating blood pressure.

Adrenal Fatigue and Stress Syndrome

Stress is the cause of many modern day disease states. Hans Selye, born in 1907 in Vienna, is considered the father of the stress syndrome. He coined the term stress, or "General Adaptation Syndrome" (shortened to G.A.S.) to describe a series of events that occur in animals and humans in response to extreme stimuli.

His "Three Stages of Stress" are still used today as a standard of diagnostics and treatment for stress-related disorders.

The initial phase of G.A.S. is the Alarm Reaction.

This is the fight or flight reaction that most are familiar with when discussing the adrenal glands. In response to external stimuli, the adrenal glands produce cortisol and adrenaline. In an ideal situation, at that point, we either fight to defend ourselves, or we flee the situation, resolving the problem and becoming safe once again. This primordial survival defense mechanism was well suited until modern times, when stressful, or seemingly unsafe, situations became the consistent norm rather than the occasional event.

Now, professional athletes such as MMA (mixed martial arts) fighters can put their systems through amazing amounts of stress everyday, just trying not to get hit or choked out. Whereas, someone at a stressful job can spend 8 hours stressing at work and then come home and still experience stress just thinking about it.

External stimuli can be in one of four forms:

Physical: These involve working long hours, training for a big game, repetitive work in a factory, injury, and all physical trauma.
Chemical: These may be nutritional in nature, for example, eating too much sugar and too many refined and processed foods or consuming excessive alcohol; these may also be cigarette smoke, recreational drugs, airborne pollutants, poisons in our environment etc.

Thermal: These involve overheating or overcooling. Persons with low adrenal output are overly sensitive to changes in temperature and feel best in a moderate, temperate climate with few fluctuations.

Emotional: These involve lack of self-esteem, abusive situations, unfulfilled dreams, financial difficulties, parenting, death of a loved one, marriage, divorce etc. In the case of emotional stress, every event creates a stressful stimulus in the hypothalamus that creates an adrenal response.

It is important to note that the hypothalamus-adrenal response will occur whether the situation is real or perceived. In other words, our thoughts and emotions are as strong a stimulus to initiate cortisol production as the slamming of our car brakes at a busy intersection. The hypothalamus makes no discernment between these stressors.

The second stage of stress is the Resistance Stage.

The body continues its response to stress and cortisol is created in the body. Its rise and fall is the causative factor in many diseases and syndromes. At this stage, the body is still able to adapt and respond to external stimuli and to function in most situations. The adrenal glands actually hypertrophy to maintain survival, and hyperadrenia (fast adrenals) can occur if the stress is continued without relief.

The third and final stage is the Exhaustion Stage.

It is this phase where hypoadrenia (slow adrenals) becomes apparent and symptoms begin to appear.

In the Adrenal Fatigue stages, this lack of adrenal production contributes to hormonal imbalances in the reproductive cycle. The adrenal glands are the "backup" gland for the ovaries and testes, and their inability to function fully can lead to lowered levels of progesterone, testosterone, and DHEA.

How I check the adrenal glands:

1. Symptoms relating to the adrenal glands
2. Pupil response test
   I have to admit, that most of the time I use numbers 1 and 2 exclusively.
3. Postural Low Blood Pressure Test
4. Inner side knee pain   *(can use Mouth to Nerve tests)*
5. Short leg   *(can use Mouth to Nerve tests)*

1. Symptoms

The first thing I start off with is finding out if the patient has any symptoms that relate to the adrenal glands.

These are symptoms of increased cortisol from overworked

adrenal glands:

- Difficulty falling asleep, wakefulness in the night
- Reduced REM sleep
- Increased blood sugar levels
- Increased protein breakdown that can lead to muscle wasting
- Decreased immune system response (If I do blood work, I can look at the WBC count and the differentiation between white blood cells. You may see a reduced amount of Neutrophils and an increased amount of lymphocytes)
- Water retention
- Allergies

If the stress continues and the resistance phase is maintained in the body, cortisol can begin to rise throughout the day, as well as staying high during the night. When this occurs, you can observe all of the above symptoms, plus:

- High blood pressure
- Sleep apnea
- Symptoms of hypothyroidism
- Increased fat through the torso
- Reduced insulin sensitivity
- Eventual reduction in adrenal steroid precursors
- Hyperlipidemia

As the stressors continue, an individual moves over the top of the sine wave curve from the peak point, and cortisol begins to decline as he/she enters the exhaustion phase. At this point, cortisol output is lower than normal, and the person may exhibit a myriad of symptoms, including:

- Crashing fatigue, especially in the afternoon
- Feelings of anxiety and unreasonable tension

- Muscle and joint pain (due to the body's lack of the natural anti-inflammatory hormone, cortisol)
- Asthma or heavy chest
- Air hunger, inability to breathe deeply
- Periodic bouts of rapid heart beat
- Hot flashes or night sweats
- GI disturbances, indigestion, flatulence, bloating
- Fibromyalgia symptoms
- Inability to relax
- Insomnia, difficulty waking in morning
- Chronic back pain
- Irregular menstrual periods
- Low sex drive
- Erectile dysfunction
- PMS and cramps
- Feeling cold often
- Mental confusion or brain fog
- Allergies and sinusitis
- Depression and mood swings
- Exacerbation of existing conditions
- Alcohol intolerance
- Hypoglycemia symptoms
- Early onset of menopause
- Dizziness, lightheadedness

It is important to note how many symptoms listed above mimic other diseases. Often, a patient is diagnosed with blood sugar dysfunction, perimenopause, or another symptomatic complaint and is treated specifically for that symptom. The patient will typically not get very good results because they are not being treated for the underlying condition, which is an adrenal gland problem.

The patient or athlete may complain of chronic knee pain or low back pain, due to the association of the sartorius, gracilis, gastrocnemius, soleus, and tibialis posterior muscles. These muscles can weaken with adrenal exhaustion and knee stability will decrease. Vulnerability to injury, tripping, frequent accidents, and lack of awareness of their surroundings may be observed.

2. Pupil Response Test

a. Do this in a room that is not bright with light because you do not want the pupil to start in a constricted position. It is easiest to do the test in a low light room because the patient's pupils will be open to allow more light in.

b. Shine a penlight at the pupil in a 45-degree angle.

c. Watch what happens to the pupil.

Here is what happens and how to evaluate what you see:

Perfect: pupil constricts and holds tight for 15 seconds without pulsing

Ok: pupil constricts and holds tight for 10 seconds before pulsing

Needs support: pupil pulses right away and becomes larger before 10 seconds

Needs a lot of support: pupil doesn't constrict or barely constricts. (This could also be from some type of nerve or brain problem or drugs)

3. Postural Low Blood Pressure Test

(This test is a little more advanced. You have to have a blood pressure cuff and know how to use it)

A measurable sign of adrenal exhaustion is Postural Hypotension, determined by measuring blood pressure.

Ideally, when a person rises from supine (laying on your back face up) position to standing, there is a rise of 8 mm mercury in the systolic reading.

In the weak adrenal patient, the comparative blood pressure reading will actually be lower by several points when tested standing after being tested lying down.

a. Lay down on your back.

b. Put blood pressure cuff on and determine the systolic pressure.

c. Pump up the cuff again while you are still laying down to 15-25 mm/Hg above what is was on the first measurement. Then stand up quickly.

d. Determine the systolic pressure within 5 seconds of standing up.

Here is what happens and how to evaluate the test:

Perfect: 8-10 point rise in systolic pressure when you stand up

Ok: systolic pressure stays the same when you stand up

Needs support: systolic pressure drops when you stand up

Needs a lot of support: systolic pressure drops over 15 points when you stand up. You may even get dizzy when standing up.

Mouth to Nerve tests (doctors commonly call this Neuro-Lingual taste testing)

Neuro-Lingual taste testing can be utilized with these tests: the inner side knee pain and short leg tests.

This is what you do. 1. Do the test 2. Then put a nutrient in your mouth resting on the tongue 3. Then re-evaluate the test.

If the results improve, the nutrient should help the adrenal glands. If the test gets worse, the nutrient will not be beneficial. You can test one nutrient at a time or a combination of nutrients.

Between each nutrient test, you will need to spit out the nutrient and rinse your mouth out with water.

Just so you are aware of this, there are also lab tests to evaluate adrenal function. For instance, cortisol and DHEA are commonly looked at. I also like to look at the potassium level in the blood. I compare results to a perfect blood potassium level of 4.0 to 4.5.

The adrenal glands push potassium into the cell. If the blood level is 4.6 and above, that is an indicator that the adrenal glands are underperforming and are not pushing enough potassium into the cells. This would likely be from a person who is burned out (exhaustion phase). So I would give them supplements such as adrenal glandulars for support.

If the blood level was 3.9 or below, I would say that the adrenals are overworking (resistance phase) and I would recommend adaptagen herbs to help the body adapt to stress. I also recommend drinking a superfood smoothie daily, because the superfoods help your body adapt to stress.

4. Inner side knee pain

Push on the inner side (medial) of your knee and note how tender it is. The more pain, the more adrenal stress.

(You can test nutrients on inner side knee pain by using the mouth to nerve test explained above. When putting a beneficial nutrient in your mouth on your tongue, the tenderness will decrease)

5. Short Leg

This is a test that many doctors use that takes a bit of practice. I know that at first I questioned what I was looking at, initially, but now it is so easy for me that it is second nature.

This test cannot be done on yourself. The person being tested must lay face down and have their head in a neutral position. It also helps to have a massage or chiropractic table for this. Turning the head to either side can throw off the test because doing so is an indicator for neck problems.

The person doing the testing will look down and see if one leg is short. It helps to wear shoes and line up the soles.

Some people have an actual short leg that is not short from the adrenal glands. For instance, they broke their leg and now that leg is short. This is not a good test for these types of people. However, you can look at the relative change from the initial starting point.

(You can test nutrients with the short leg test by using the mouth to nerve test explained above. When putting a beneficial nutrient in your mouth on your tongue, the short leg will become even in length with the longer leg. If the short leg becomes even shorter when the substance is placed in the mouth, that substance should be avoided)

After testing a nutrient, have the patient stand and take a few steps then lay back down. This acts to reset the pelvic and postural muscles. Also, rinse your mouth out with water between testing each nutrient.

An Acidic pH is a problem

Another commonly overlooked point is that being overly acidic can cause the adrenal glands to be hyper (overactive). It is important to increase fruits, vegetables and superfood smoothies, which are alkaline. Taking the minerals magnesium and zinc, which are alkaline, can also help. Sugar is also very acidic, so reducing sugar intake can be beneficial.

Superfoods are effective to support hormones and glands

When we started formulating the superfood mixes for My Nutrition Advisor, we wanted one mix to provide support to the endocrine (glands and hormones) system. As it turned out, all the superfood mixes have ingredients that provide support. I have noticed that the Ancient Chocolate mix has excelled at providing support for hormonal problems.

I have the unique opportunity of seeing high-level professional athletes who commonly stress out their adrenal glands from extreme amounts of exercise. Over the last year, my recommendations have been to consume to 2 to 4 tablespoons per day of Ancient Chocolate superfood mix. This is the most effective method of using food to support the adrenal glands that I have used to date.

26 What is a Superfood?

The complete definition of "Superfood" is not universally agreed upon. However, what is agreed upon is that certain foods have much higher nutrition levels than other foods.

We can also agree that some foods have a much higher antioxidant count than other foods, which can quench harmful free radicals.

Lastly, we can agree that some foods have tendencies to prevent certain medical problems.

As an example, let's look at two fruits:

1. Acerola cherries are considered a superfood.

2. Oranges are not considered a superfood.

It is easy to see why one is considered a superfood and one is not. Compare the nutrient levels between these two.

One cup of oranges contains 95 mg of vitamin C. Once cup of acerola cherries contain 1644 mg of vitamin C. Wow, what a difference! When we compare other nutrients, acerola cherries provide double the amount of potassium, magnesium and pantothenic acid as oranges.

27 Let Your Food Be Your Medicine

Here is what you may or may not realize yet: What you put in your mouth has much more of a direct influence on your overall health than you have been lead to realize.

If you regularly drink sodas and eat processed foods, you will NOT have optimal health. When you buy the popular mass marketed junk food that many people eat daily, you are destroying your health.

The miracle is what you eat, not a pill:

People run off to their doctors wanting to get a medicine that will magically make them healthy. However, this magical medicine does not exist. Can prescription drugs help certain conditions? Yes. However, prescription drugs do not magically give you optimal health. Your doctor knows this very well and this is why your doctor has recommended to you to completely change your diet to natural foods.

Unless you change what you eat and what you feed your kids, you and your kids will not have optimal health.

Bad Strategy:

If you eat nothing but processed junk food and drink soda for every meal, you will likely have a bunch of health problems such as diabetes, high blood pressure, high cholesterol, depression, sleep apnea, digestion problems, constipation and hormone problems.

Good Strategy:

Superfoods actually improve your health and give your body the nutrients it needs to work properly. Superfoods prevent and/or improve many chronic health problems and everyone should be informed of this.

What are some of the most potent superfoods and why do we use them?

In this section, I decided not to list every piece of research on each superfood as there is simply way too much for this book to hold. If you would like to see research, you can go to pubmed.gov and do searches for these superfoods. There are hundreds of studies and every month the count grows larger. To save space, I am going to list some high points on each of the following superfoods, rather than quote each study.

I chose to write about some of my favorite superfoods that I used to formulate the CappuGreeno and Superfood Smoothie mixes for My Nutrition Advisor.

Acai Berries – Native to the Amazon rainforest region and nicknamed the "Beauty Berry." The Acai berry packs a huge amount of nutritional value. Acai berries contain very high antioxidant properties and are used for various health conditions – including high cholesterol, weight loss, detoxification, and for improving general health.

Acerola Cherries - A West Indian cherry that serves as one of the richest sources of Vitamin C. Acerola cherries have high antioxidant properties and are commonly used as a natural remedy for numerous health conditions – including high blood sugar, stress, heart disease, and cancer. They are also used to promote healthy toned skin and youthful appearance.

Beet Root - One of the richest dietary sources of antioxidants and naturally occurring nitrates. Nitrates are compounds, which improve blood flow throughout the body – including the brain, heart, and muscles. They naturally support detoxification, circulation / blood pressure, energy production, stamina, and nitric oxide levels. Beet fiber provides the benefit of protecting us from colon cancer.

Cacao – Is the bean that comes from the cacao tree in raw form. Once it is roasted and processed it is called cocoa. It has been an important South American food for thousands of years. Cacao is packed with natural antioxidants, magnesium and iron. Cacao is associated with many benefits such as stress relief, improving depression and heart function. It has also been used to support circulation and lower blood pressure. Cacao helps our brains create anandamide, also known as the "Bliss Chemical".

Camu Camu - Grown in the Amazon rain forest, this fruit's leaves contain more vitamin C than any other plant in the world, which is 30 to 60 times more than an orange! It is known as a potent anti-viral compound. It is also known to boost energy, provide immune system support, fight inflammation, and reduce stress.

Chia Seeds, Flax Seeds, Hemp Seeds - Originating from different areas of the world, these super seeds provide concentrated sources of healthy fatty acids (omegas), amino acids, protein, and fiber. They are commonly used for appetite suppression, skin problems and digestion support including constipation. Evidence suggests that they can lower the risk of diabetes, cancer and heart disease.

Cinnamon - It has a very long history being used as both a spice and a medicine. It was mentioned in the Bible and was used in ancient Egypt. It is also mentioned in Chinese medicine books around 2700 B.C.

Here are some of the health related things cinnamon has been used for:

Blood sugar support: The American Journal of Clinical Nutrition reported that participants given rice pudding with three grams of cinnamon produced less insulin after a meal. Cinnamon also slows the rate at which food leaves the stomach after a meal. This keeps you satisfied longer after a meal. In another study, it was shown that consuming as little as one gram of cinnamon per day was found to reduce blood sugar, triglycerides and bad cholesterol.

Anti-Microbial: It is used to stop growth of bacteria and fungi including Candida.

Anti-Clotting: It has been used to prevent unwanted blood platelet clumping.

Antioxidant and skin health: It contains antioxidants that protect against oxidation. Cinnamon also contains various phenols that help protect against advanced glycation end-products (AGEs), which cause tissue damage, inflammation, visible lines on the face and inflexible arteries.

Brain Function: Just smelling cinnamon increases brain function.

It is also a source of fiber and the minerals manganese, iron and calcium.

Coconut Palm Sugar - A low glycemic neutral sweetener that has been used for thousands of years in Asia. It produces a steady, slow energy release while also providing a high amount of essential minerals.

Ginger - It has long been used for cooking and as an herbal medicine. The Romans imported ginger from China approximately 2000 years ago.

It is commonly given to relieve gastrointestinal stress, including gas and spasms. Ginger is also given for motion sickness. It has antioxidant and anti-inflammatory effects. People use ginger to reduce arthritic pain.

Another use of ginger is to support the immune system and provide additional support to cancer patients.

Many pregnant women use ginger to reduce nausea and vomiting.

Goji Berries - A nutritionally rich fruit native to China that has been used in traditional Chinese Medicine for thousands of years. It is packed with vitamins, minerals, protein and antioxidants. It contains 21 trace minerals, including germanium, which is rarely found in foods. Goji berries also contain more beta-carotene than carrots and zeaxanthin, which protects the eyes. It is known to support brain function, cardiovascular health, joint health, endurance, energy and anti-aging.

Lucuma - "The Gold of the Incas", this ancient Peruvian superfruit is a low glycemic natural sweetener that is also an excellent source of antioxidants, fiber, vitamins, and 14 essential minerals. It has both anti-inflammatory and anti-oxidant properties. Lucuma is also believed to help with wound healing and skin aging.

Maca Root - It is a root from the radish family that is legendary for naturally increasing energy and stamina. It is rich in vitamins, minerals, enzymes and amino acids. It is a vegetarian source of B12 and also contains very useable forms of calcium and magnesium.

It has been used traditionally to balance hormones by nourishing the glands of the body. It is a strong adaptogen, which means it helps you to individually adapt to your own bodies needs. In other words if you are producing too little of a hormone it helps you produce more and if you are producing too much of a hormone, it helps to down regulate production.

It is equally effective with men and women. It is a staple food from the high mountains of Peru and is also used to help with a range of things from menopause and mood balance to libido. It is also commonly taken for skin issues.

Maqui Berries - A treasure from the Mapuche Indians of southern Chile, who are the only indigenous people in the Americas who have never been conquered by an invading force. The Mapuche have used the Maqui berry for both food and medicine for centuries.

Maqui berries have extremely high antioxidant levels such as anthocyanins, delphinidin, malvidin, petunidin, cumarins, triterpenes, flavanoids and cyaniding. They have the highest ORAC levels of any fruit, which are approximately four times higher than blueberries and twice as high as acai berries.

They are also a good source of vitamin C, calcium, potassium and iron. Maqui berries support the cardiovascular system by encouraging blood flow and are also used for inflammation.

Moringa - "The Miracle Tree", native to parts of Africa and Asia, is considered by many to be one of the most complete, nutrient-rich trees on Earth. For instance, moringa leaves contain: four times the calcium as milk, three times the potassium of bananas, four times the vitamin A of carrots, seven times the vitamin C of oranges and two times the protein of yogurt.

Moringa has been used around the world for inflammation, diabetes, iron deficiency, high blood pressure, and healthy joints.

Pomegranate - One of the oldest known fruits, pomegranate originated from the Mediterranean and is a nutrient dense, antioxidant rich fruit that has been revered as a symbol of health, fertility, and eternal life. It is thought to provide many health benefits including cardiovascular health, cancer fighter, cholesterol fighter, and immune system booster. Pomegranate has been shown to elevate the major antioxidant produced in the liver called glutathione.

Reishi Mushroom - This Asian bioactive fungus is well known for boosting the immune system. It is also used for viral, fungal and yeast infections, lung conditions, heart disease, high blood pressure, high cholesterol, cancer, fatigue, sleep, stress, and to help maintain blood glucose levels.

Spirulina - Used as a food source since the 9th century. These freshwater blue-green algae are believed to help stimulate the immune system, increase production of antibodies, protect against liver damage, have antiviral and anticancer properties as well as support the development of red blood cells.

They consist of 60% protein and are considered a complete protein because they contain all 22 essential amino acids. Spirulina also contains a large amount of vitamins, minerals, antioxidants, phytonutrients and chlorophyll. They are one of the few plant sources of vitamin B12.

Turmeric Root – An orange colored root that is related to ginger. It contains a powerful antioxidant and anti-inflammatory compound called curcumin.

You may be familiar with turmeric because it is the ingredient in curry that gives curry its color and distinctive flavor.

While doing research on Alzheimer's disease, it was noticed that this disease was four times lower in India, where curry is eaten, compared to rates in the United States. Researchers believed that the turmeric, in the curry, was responsible for the lower rates of Alzheimer's disease in India.

Later research showed that this belief turned out to be true. The curcumin in the turmeric actually helps inhibit the accumulation of harmful beta amyloids in the brain. Curcumin also helps inhibit inflammation in the brain, which is common with Alzheimer's disease as well as inflammation around the rest of the body.

This is why doctors around the world use turmeric to treat conditions that have an inflammation component, such as arthritis.

The really exciting thing about turmeric is that it has been shown to influence more than 700 genes in your body. This is the reason that anti-aging doctors started recommending turmeric to "slow" the aging process and prevent diseases such as cancer and diabetes.

Curcumin has also been shown to hold back fat accumulation.

Wheatgrass - A nutrient-rich type of young grass in the wheat family that contains a variety of nutrients, which are used to detoxify and alkalize your blood. It also contains chlorophyll, which helps form red blood cells and oxygenates your blood. Although wheat is in the name, it does not contain gluten.

28 STOP GETTING SICK SO MUCH

The most effective ways to strengthen your immune system are to make sure you are doing these things:

1. Eat plenty of superfoods
2. Get enough sleep
3. Get sunlight or take vitamin D
4. Get some exercise.

Overall, the equation is pretty simple. Do these things and your immune system will be significantly stronger than if you don't.

No medications for 25 years

I frequently get questions about what to give sick kids. When I look on facebook, I see a lot of posts about sick kids. Some of the posts even talk about the stuff parents are giving their kids, like over-the-counter cold remedies from the grocery store etc. My personal thoughts on these cold remedies are that they are not only harmful to your kids, but they prolong the illness. Do your own research.

Just so you know where I am coming from, my 15 year old has never taken a medication, such as an antibiotic, nor has he taken a cold remedy that is designed to cover up symptoms. It is now 2014 and the last time I took a medication was 1989 when I got food poisoning while in college.

I have used many vitamins, minerals, herbs, spices etc. over the years to keep my immune system strong. I am not saying medications don't have a place, I am saying that they are widely overused and often cause more problems than they help.

My kids enjoy a superfood smoothie when they come home from school.

This one simple step makes a huge difference in their health. Their favorite recipes are:

Mint Chocolate Chunk, Hawaiian Greens, Pumpkin Peanut Butter Cup, Peanut Butter and Jelly, Heirloom Pear, Red Velvet Cupcake and Salted Chocolate Caramel.

In the fall, winter and spring months, my kids take vitamin D. I give them each 2000 iu per day. There is a lot of research on having optimal blood levels of vitamin D for the immune system to work properly. Some researches have come out and said that vitamin D is very important to prevent the flu.

So what happens if we get sick?

Everyone gets sick now and then, but it is usually not necessary to take antibiotics for the typical cold. As a doctor myself, I have found that the strategies below work very well.

If anyone comes down with a cold in my family, we immediately do a couple things.

1. Take oregano essential oil and thieves essential oil, a few to several times, each day until the cold is gone. We usually take 1 – 4 drops per meal of oregano essential oil. Oregano essential oil burns, so I drop it onto the food that is already in my mouth to mask the burning effect. Thieves essential oil is much easier to take as I rub it on my throat, feet and drop it in my mouth. If I wake up with a sore throat in the middle of the night, I put a few drops of thieves essential oil directly onto my tongue and go back to sleep.
2. We rub thieves essential oil on the bottom of our feet when we go to bed.
3. We drink a superfood smoothie everyday using the Ancient Delight superfood mix from My Nutrition Advisor. This mix is geared towards supporting the immune system.

29 High Blood Pressure and Type 2 Diabetes Protocols

I seriously debated putting these protocols in this book. Sometimes old memories of being attacked die-hard. When I had a radio show, 15 years ago, I did several shows on blood pressure and type 2 diabetes. I was frequently invited to give presentations on these topics and a few times spoke to pretty large groups.

I helped a lot of people get to the point where they no longer required medications for high blood pressure and type 2 diabetes. However, I was warned that giving people solutions to help them with these problems, without using drugs, is a potential violation and I could lose my license.

I even had a fellow chiropractor come to my office and tell me that I should no longer help people with high blood pressure because it was bad for chiropractors to do anything other than treat back and neck pain. I told this doctor that I was using nutrition to get at the cause of the problem. He felt that was wrong and I should not be using nutrition and I should not help people fix their problems other than joint and nerve pain. I even shared with him many patient testimonials of great successes. At that time I had over 100 patient success testimonials for high blood pressure and type 2 diabetes. Apparently that wasn't good enough and he said that these people should be only treated with drugs.

This was around 1999 and information wasn't readily available all over the internet as it is today. Most of my patients didn't even have the internet yet for that matter. The only time I drew more heat was when I did some radio shows on the dangers of GMOs and asked listeners to call their politicians to vote against GMOs when Clinton was president. That is a whole other story that caused me tons of problems for being one of the first in the country to speak out against GMOs.

When it comes to high blood pressure and type 2 diabetes, I tell patients to discuss the protocols with their doctor and work with their doctor to reduce their prescription medication as needed. For instance, when one starts to follow the type 2 diabetes protocols, their blood sugar typically drops and they need to reduce the dosage of their medications. (Isn't that obvious?)

However, when I said it 15 years ago on the radio, I was attacked and criticized pretty hard. Fast-forward to now; studies have been performed that say exactly what I was saying in the late 1990s. It is not always good to be a pioneer. You usually get attacked and then others come behind you later on to get all the credit and find a way to make money off of it.

With that being said, here are my protocols. I group these two protocols together because I have found that that overall, the basis of the protocols are similar and only a few minor steps are different.

Blood Pressure and Type 2 Diabetes:

1. How often you eat and what you eat are the biggest deciding factors for blood pressure and type 2 diabetes. If you choose to ignore these factors, you have no one to blame but yourself.

2. Eat 2 to 3 times per day. Preferably twice. Make these two meals as close to each other as possible. I call this eating in a window. Let's say you eat lunch at noon and then dinner at 6 PM. You have just eaten in a 6-hour window. I recommend a six to eight hour window.

3. Fast when you are not in the window. That means that you will not eat or drink anything with calories during this time. So if your window is from noon to 6 PM, do not eat from 6:01 PM until noon the next day.

    This fasting time does some very important things. Fasting decreases insulin, which decreases the fluid volume in your body. A higher fluid volume increases blood pressure. By decreasing insulin levels, your cells become more sensitive to insulin, which helps to more effectively lower blood sugar levels.

Eating frequently and eating lots of sugar is the fastest way to increase insulin levels. So I would suggest that you don't do either as increased insulin levels lead to higher fluid volume quickly and higher blood sugar levels over time. Sugar makes you thirsty because it stimulates insulin. When you have a higher level of insulin in your blood, you will retain a large amount of the fluid you drink in your blood vessels. This increase in fluid will raise your blood pressure.

4. Drink a Superfood Smoothie for one meal per day. The superfood mixes from My Nutrition Advisor contain ingredients that help circulation as well as many other functions. See the chapters on "Raising Nitric Oxide" and "What is a Superfood". For instance, the superfoods beet and cacao are valuable to eat for blood pressure, while cinnamon, chia, flax and hemp seeds are valuable to eat for type 2 diabetes.

> I have done blood pressure testing and blood sugar testing before and after eating many types of meals. The best results that I have been able to obtain with patients and with myself is with superfood smoothies. I believe these are the most effective meals one can consume based off what I have seen with actual testing.

5. Eat "healthy" food at your other meal. This will preferably be a meal with plenty of vegetables as the main ingredients. Foods to avoid are anything processed. That includes processed meats, grains and foods full of artificial stuff. Limit baked goods like pastas, breads, and cakes. Avoid fast foods and sodas as well. For the most part, vegetables cause a low insulin response, while processed and baked foods cause a high insulin response.

6. Take magnesium for both high blood pressure and type 2 diabetes. Think of it this way: Magnesium relaxes muscles and calcium contracts muscles. If the muscles around your arteries are contracted, your blood pressure will be elevated. I have been doing blood tests for many years and it is way more common to be deficient in magnesium than calcium. You can really see the difference on micronutrient blood tests that look into cells rather than standard serum tests.

If you go to the hospital with really high blood pressure, they will give you an IV with magnesium. So if a person is given an IV with magnesium at the hospital, it will relax the muscles in their blood vessels. This dilates the blood vessels, which lowers blood pressure. It should be noted that it could be dangerous to give magnesium in an IV because if it is given too quickly it can stop the heart. When taken orally, it takes time for the magnesium to absorb. Some doctors keep liquid magnesium chloride in their offices to give to patients with high blood pressure because it absorbs much quicker than magnesium pills. However, magnesium chloride tastes terrible.

Here are the dosing guidelines for magnesium pills. Take around 600 mg per day on an empty stomach. If you take too much, you will get diarrhea and should take less the next day. By the way, this symptom of diarrhea also applies to vitamin C. Some people step their dosage up 1 pill per day until they get loose stools and then back off 1 pill the next day. This way they keep themselves at the maximum dosage they can absorb.

The forms that work best are magnesium chloride, magnesium orotate, magnesium gluconate, and magnesium glycinate. The form to avoid because of poor absorption is magnesium oxide. It is important to take magnesium on an empty stomach. If you take it with food, it will bind to the fat that you eat and be lost in the feces. Cheap fat blocker products use magnesium oxide to bind to the fats eaten. If the magnesium is bound to the eaten fats, it will not benefit you because it is not being absorbed.

It should be noted that people with certain conditions are best to avoid certain things. Such as someone with Renal (Kidney) insufficiency should avoid taking magnesium. This is why it is recommended to consult with your doctor before starting to take supplements. At least, do a web search and look this stuff up for yourself.

7. Take Fish oil, as it has been shown to help lipid (fat) metabolism and insulin sensitivity. I generally recommend 5000 mg per day for patients with high blood pressure and type 2 diabetes.

8. Take 4000 iu of Vitamin D per day or get sun exposure daily. I use this for high blood pressure and type 2 diabetes.

9. Take CoQ-10 for both high blood pressure and type 2 diabetes. I generally recommend 100 mg with two meals per day.

These last three ingredients below, I recommend for Type 2 Diabetes.

10. Take Chromium and Vanadium. They are minerals that help with blood sugar. I generally recommend sources from vegetable cultures, as they seem to work the best. The dosages I recommend are 200 mcg of chromium with two meals per day and 20 mcg of vanadium with two meals per day.

11. Take Alpha-Lipoic Acid. It is an antioxidant that helps with blood sugar by improving insulin sensitivity. I generally recommend 100 mg with two meals per day.

30 Questions for Weight Loss

This section will assist you in evaluating the best methods and techniques to aid in you in your weight loss goals. (Be honest. You are only harming yourself if you aren't truthful in your answers.)

It is important to realize that weight loss comes down to how many calories you consume compared to how many calories your body needs to function. When you create a deficit of calories from what your body needs, you will lose fat.

The most important question to ask is how can you drop the

calories you are consuming so that you create a deficit in a way that you will stick with. This is the million-dollar question.

This is also why I strongly recommend you read my book *Fat Loss The Truth*. I cover what the research says works and I also speak from the experience of seeing over 5000 weight loss clients. If a person really wants to lose weight, it is extremely beneficial to learn the medical truths and use strategies that have actually been researched. Anyone can give weight loss advice, but I give advice that people actually stick with in *Fat Loss The Truth*.

How to use this chapter

Answer the questions below to see what methods you can choose to help you reach your goals. If you answer yes to a question in a category, simply follow the suggested strategy.

Category 1 Appetite Suppression

1. Do you have issues eating too much when you eat?
2. Are you excessively hungry between meals?

If you answered yes, and you feel that this is something you need support for, follow the strategies in the chapter titled "Appetite Suppression".

Category 2 Cold Metabolism Stimulation

This category utilizes ice packs.

Did you know that exercising in the cold causes you to burn more calories than exercising in the heat?

Most people do not realize that there are two main types of fat. Brown adipose tissue (BAT), which burns calories, and white adipose tissue (WAT), which stores calories. We obviously want more BAT, which burns calories. Brown adipose tissue does this by converting calories into heat.

This means that when we are cold, our bodies have to convert calories into heat to warm us.

It had previously been believed that the brown fat found in infants disappears as we grow up, but the latest information shows that this is not the case. Brown fat cells have been found in adults, in the lower part of the neck just above the collarbone. (By placing cold ice packs in this area, we stimulate the brown fat to burn calories. This is an additional way to require your body to burn more calories)

This strategy of using cold metabolism therapy focuses on increasing the amount of calories burned by the brown fat cells.

The easiest way to start to use cold metabolism therapy is to place ice packs above your collarbones for 30 minutes per day. Exercising in the cold for 20 minutes at a time is another complimentary strategy. Swimming in cool water is the fastest way to burn calories.

Category 3 Detoxification and Inflammation

1. Do you commonly have incomplete digestion of your food?

2. Do you commonly get constipated?
3. Do you commonly have diarrhea?
4. Are you frequently bloated?
5. Are you sensitive to several different foods?
6. Do you have frequent body aches and pains?
7. Do you have frequent skin outbreaks?
8. Do you have frequent stiffness in your joints?

If you answered yes, and you feel that this is something you need support for, follow the strategies in the chapters titled "5-Day Detoxification Plan" and "A Constipation Fix".

Category 4 Endurance and Energy Production

1. Do you have low energy levels?
2. Do you get worn out and tired easy?
3. Do your muscles get easily fatigued?
4. Do you feel exhausted after moderate exercise?
5. Do you frequently consume soda?
6. Do you frequently consume processed junk foods?
7. Do you eat less than 8 servings of vegetables per day?

If you answered yes, and you feel that this is something you need support for, follow the strategies in the chapters titled "Raising Nitric Oxide" and "Are You Tired After Lunch?"

Category 5 Fat Burning Supplements

1. Do you feel caffeine is beneficial for you without causing you to become jittery?

If you answered yes, and you feel that this is something you need support for, follow the strategies in the chapter titled "Coffee and CappuGreeno Recipes".

Category 6 Gut Microbes

1. Have you taken antibiotics and not replaced the good bacteria (i.e. flora) afterwards with a supplement?
2. Do you commonly use artificial sweeteners such as sucralose?

If you answered yes, I would recommend making Superfood Smoothies that contain strawberries and/or a banana in the recipes. Yogurt is another ingredient that can be beneficial if it contains probiotics. I also recommend taking a probiotic supplement for at least a couple months.

Category 7 Hormone Support

1. Do you feel like your sex hormones are low?
2. Is your sex drive low?
3. Are you suffering from menopause?

One of the most effective superfoods to support hormones is maca. Maca is discussed in the chapter titled "Let Your Food be Your Medicine". It is in the superfood mixes from My Nutrition Advisor called Ancient Chocolate, Ancient Delight and Ancient Greens. If you answered yes, I would recommend that you consume superfood smoothies with one of these three superfood mixes that contain maca. I also recommend taking a supplement that contains velvet antler for both men and women. There is a big difference between velvet antler supplements, so don't go for the cheap one. You will typically get what you pay for.

4. Do you feel that your thyroid gland is slow? (e.g. slow metabolism)
5. Are you commonly cold?
6. Has the outer 1/3 of your eyebrows disappeared?

These questions relate to the thyroid gland. If you answered yes, and you feel that this is something you need support for, follow the strategies in the chapter titled "Adrenal Gland Tests". The reason I suggest to read this chapter is because the adrenal glands and thyroid gland work closely together. Providing support to the adrenal glands frequently benefits the thyroid as well.

To support the thyroid gland, one should choose superfood smoothie recipes that contain sea salt to add specific nourishment to the thyroid gland. Sea salt contains a large variety of trace minerals and other major minerals that are necessary for thyroid function. One specific recipe that I recommend frequently is called Salted Chocolate Caramel and can be found on the My Nutrition Advisor website.

Re-read the chapter "High Blood Pressure and Type 2 Diabetes Protocols". This chapter contains a section about taking magnesium, which is essential to the thyroid gland. I would suggest taking supplemental magnesium as well.

Lastly, I would recommend taking iodine to feed the thyroid. This is something that you should ask your doctor for recommendations before you start taking. The common supplement used by doctors contains 5 mg of Iodine and 7.5 mg of Potassium Iodide per tablet and I usually recommend one tablet per day.

7. Do you crave sweets?
8. Do you have fatigue that is relieved by eating?
9. Do you have excessive thirst?

If you answered yes, and you feel that this is something you need support for, follow the strategies in the chapter titled "Blood Sugar Home Testing".

10. Do you feel burned out?
11. Are you commonly feeling stressed?
12. Do you commonly feel anxiety?
13. Are you a worrier?
14. Do you have feelings of insecurity?
15. Are your eyes sensitive to the sun or lights at night?
16. Are you a slow starter in the morning?
17. Are you calm on the outside and troubled on the inside?
18. Are you frequently dizzy when standing up suddenly?
19. Do you have difficulty falling asleep?
20. Do you tend to be a night person?

If you answered yes, and you feel that this is something you need support for, follow the strategies in the chapter titled "Adrenal Gland Tests".

21. Do you have arthritic tendencies?

If you answered yes, I would consume one to two superfood smoothies per day. I would also focus on recipes that contain cherries.

Category 8 Hypnosis

This category does not utilize smoothies but instead uses hypnosis tapes.

Hypnosis is a tool that can make everything you do easier and more effective. It is most beneficial when it is added to any weight loss and weight management plan as the studies below indicate.

Surveying the results of hypnosis combined with a sensible weight loss program proved that including hypnosis improved the effectiveness of the weight loss program by an AVERAGE OF 97% while being treated, and improved the effectiveness AFTER TREATMENT by a whopping 146%! (Journal of Consulting and Clinical Psychology, 1996).

One study divided a group of sixty women into two groups; one group received hypnotherapy for weight loss and the other received no hypnotherapy. Suffice it to say that the group receiving hypnotherapy lost an average of 17lbs while the group that went without hypnotherapy only 1/2 pound on average! (Journal of Consulting and Clinical Psychology, 1986).

In a different study that followed two different weight loss programs for 9 weeks, the group that received hypnotherapy was STILL getting results when the researchers followed up two-years later while the group that went without hypnotherapy had no further progress (Journal of Clinical Psychology, 1985).

Did you know these nuggets of hypnosis history?
These little-known hypnosis success stories may just inspire you too. Most people never learned these facts in school!
1. Sir Winston Churchill used post hypnotic suggestions to stay refreshed even though he was up all night during much of World War 2.
2. Tiger Woods used hypnosis to help him block out distractions and achieve laser-focus on the golf course.
3. Wolfgang Mozart composed his famous opera "Cosi fan tutte" while in a hypnotic trance!
4. Steve Hooker of Australia won the 2008 Gold Medal in Pole Vaulting after hypnosis helped him visualize winning.
5. Albert Einstein's Theory of Relativity came to him during one of his daily hypnosis sessions.
6. Mike Tyson used extensive amounts of hypnosis while rising to the top and maintaining the heavyweight boxing title.

But how can you experience the phenomenal results of hypnosis... without paying an arm and a leg for professional hypnotherapy sessions?
www.Hypfit.net

Simply listen to a session in your iPod every night when you go to bed. It helps you get to sleep and only takes 8 to 20 minutes per session.

31 Start Today -Fat Loss Guide –

1. Start with a 5-day detoxification plan
2. Eat all food for the day in a 6-hour window of time
3. Upon completion of the 5-day detoxification plan, eat one superfood smoothie and one meal per day in the 6-hour window
4. Take a good fat burner and multi-vitamin/ or targeted supplements.
5. Read Fat Loss The Truth

1. Start with a 5-day detoxification plan.

- Cleaning toxins out of your body puts you into a fat burning mode.
- Superfoods contain nutrients that promote detoxification.
- Drink 24 – 48 ounces of superfood smoothies per day to get enough cleansing superfoods into your system. Do not eat regular food during the 5-day detoxification.

(Many people immediately feel more energy and start to sleep better. However, some people may not feel great during the intense 5-day detoxification. Remember, your body will be cleaning itself at a fast rate. If it becomes too intense, simply reduce the detoxification rate by drinking one 24-ounce smoothie per day and have 1 healthy meal per day that is preferably vegetable soup and a salad)

2. **Eat all food for the day in a 6-hour window of time.**

   - Your organs detoxify your body when you are in a fasted state.
   - Twelve hours after you eat, your body speeds up detoxifying itself and burning fat for energy.
   - Eating all your food for the day in a 6-hour window, gives your body 18 hours to detoxify and burn fat for energy.

   Pick times that work for you:
   Example: Consume a superfood smoothie at noon and then consume another superfood smoothie at 6 PM.

Common Problem: If you eat when you first wake-up in the morning (7AM) and right before you go to bed (10 PM), your body does not have much time to detoxify itself. (9 total hours).

You will not reach the time period where your body starts to intensely detoxify itself and burn fat for energy.

3. **Eat one superfood smoothie and one meal per day in the 6-hour window.**

   After you have completed the 5-day detoxification plan, continue to eat in the 6-hour window.

   - Continue to benefit from fasting 18 hours per day. Your body will be detoxifying itself for many hours everyday, which allows you to burn fat each day.

   - By consuming a low calorie, filling superfood smoothie as one of your daily meals, you are only typically consuming about 200 - 400 calories for one of your meals. To put that into perspective, a 12oz glass of 2% milk is 170 calories. By consuming a low calorie, highly nutritious, and filling smoothie as one of your meals – you will feel better and have a lot more freedom to live life with your other meal.

4. **Take a good fat burner and multi-vitamin/ or targeted supplements.**

- Superfood smoothies provide more nutrition in your diet than anything else you will eat. We also recommend taking another boost of nutrients.

- Option 1: Take some type of Fat Burner supplement in the morning while you are still fasting and take a high quality multi-vitamin at dinner.

    (My Nutrition Advisor sells the fat burner supplement I currently recommend. It has ingredients that support appetite suppression, hormones, and energy in a single product that can be taken on an empty stomach during your fasting hours).

- Option 2: This involves targeted nutritional testing so you can understand your specific nutritional deficiencies and focus on supplements or vitamins to correct those deficiencies. The testing methods I utilize range from blood work micronutrient testing to biocommunication scans.

5. **Read the book *Fat Loss The Truth*.**

    It will provide you with:
    1.) A deeper understanding of how and why you are losing weight using this program.
    2.) Many tips and tricks to make your fat loss more effective and long term.

    You are committing yourself to do the first four steps; don't sell yourself short by skipping this step. What you learn can make or break your success.

    Order *Fat Loss The Truth* today and read it before next weekend. After you are done, share both of these two books with someone you know who is struggling with weight loss. You may just save their life.

Final Thoughts

1. Develop habits that are good for you. They can make your appearance youthful and your health optimal as you age or they can make your life miserable with poor health.
2. Utilize superfoods by putting them in smoothies and CappuGreenos.
3. Utilize fasting by eating fewer meals. This slows aging and makes it easier to keep your body weight in check.

ACKNOWLEDGEMENTS

Thank you to my proofreader Marco Rafalovich and my graphic designer Colton Fitzgerald.

Made in the USA
San Bernardino, CA
16 October 2014